Cbd Oil

Effective Pain Relief Without Medications

(A Beginner's Guide to Using Cbd Oil for Pain Relief and Better Health)

Matthew Hanes

Published By **Jordan Levy**

Matthew Hanes

All Rights Reserved

Cbd Oil: Effective Pain Relief Without Medications (A Beginner's Guide to Using Cbd Oil for Pain Relief and Better Health)

ISBN 978-1-9994868-8-4

No part of this guidebook shall be reproduced in any form without permission in writing from the publisher except in the case of brief quotations embodied in critical articles or reviews.

Legal & Disclaimer

The information contained in this book is not designed to replace or take the place of any form of medicine or professional medical advice. The information in this book has been provided for educational & entertainment purposes only.

The information contained in this book has been compiled from sources deemed reliable, and it is accurate to the best of the Author's knowledge; however, the Author cannot guarantee its accuracy and validity and cannot be held liable for any errors or omissions. Changes are periodically made to this book. You must consult your doctor or get professional medical advice before using any of the suggested remedies, techniques, or information in this book.

Table Of Contents

Chapter 1: What Exactly Is Cbd Oil? 1

Chapter 2: Types Of Cbd Oil 23

Chapter 3: Using Cbd Oil Against Illness . 39

Chapter 4: Using Cbd Oil To Curb Pain ... 53

Chapter 5: Using Cbd Oil For Mental
Health And Anxiety 64

Chapter 6: Cbd Oil Roundup 77

Chapter 7: What Is Cannabidiol (Cbd)? .. 87

Chapter 8: How Is Cbdmade? 106

Chapter 9: What Are Terpenes? 126

Chapter 10: Cbd For Pain Relief 144

Chapter 11: Cbd For Anxiety 159

Chapter 12: Ways To Enhance The Anti-
Anxiety Effects Of Cbd 170

Chapter 1: What Exactly Is Cbd Oil?

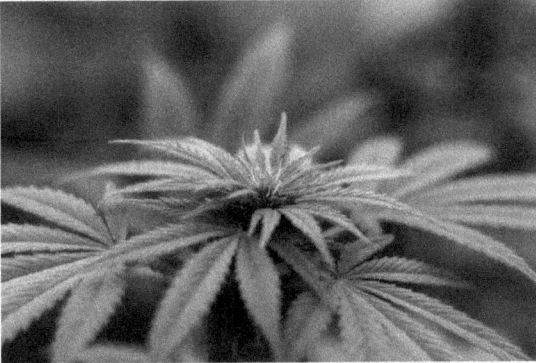

In the year 1940, an exciting discovery was made. Roger Adams, a graduate of Harvard University who would later develop into a scientist, was in obtaining cannabidiol (CBD) from Cannabis sativa. Roger Adams, at the time did not know of the significance of the results he came up with. In the time that passed, Roger Adams would eventually discover how crucial his research into CBD oil had been. He didn't work on his own or on his own in this endeavor and therefore shouldn't be considered as the sole one to have contributed to bringing the advantages of CBD oil to light.

A total of 6 years would be needed before1946 was the year the first experiment was carried out with CBD oil in lab animals. The test was carried out by Dr. Walter S. Loewe. He was Dr. Walter S. Loewe's test showed that there was no change or alteration in the mental state due to the usage of CBD oil. The same year, another test was carried out, however and this time it was done under the supervision of the Dr. Ralph Mechoulam. It was Dr. Ralph Mechoulam is often the one who gets the recognition for the discovery of CBD oil. Though he's not the first person to discover CBD oil, the Dr. Ralph Mechoulam has full credit for recognizing CBD's have a 3-dimensional design, which could pave the way for further tests as well as research being conducted by another scientist. In the early 1960s, other researchers began getting to catch up with three pioneers, Dr. Roger Adams, Dr. Walter S. Loewe, and Dr. Ralph Mechoulam as they began to study CBD oil's use in primates. After a short time, following the tests of CBD oil on primates, CBD oil was made available for use in therapeutic purposes by the British pharmaceutical firm. In the 80's the doctor. Ralph Mechoulam ran a important study which proved CBD oil was able to be used as an important factor in treatment of epilepsy. This was just the beginning of the fascinating and long story of the positive health effects of CBD oil. Since then, numerous potential benefits have been discovered as a result of its therapeutic use. as time goes on we will definitely see new discoveries and evidence of its therapeutic value coming soon.

In the present, CBD oil has a place between the it is a razor-thin line that divides debate from acceptance by the masses. In order to receive CBD oil, the product has to be obtained from hemp or marijuana. The legal system has created some barriers and hurdles that hinder CBD's increasing use widely known, well understood and recognized. The 50 United States supplements of CBD hemp-derived oil are now legally legal. It wasn't done on an easy and clear path but. There were many critics who have been averse to the inaccurate propagandistic statements and misinformation relating CBD and marijuana. CBD and CBD, all seeking to maintain CBD kept in a cage of fear and demonization. In 2014, it was reported that the United States showed a sweeping shift in culture and mentality when a number of states cleared the way for passing legislation that permitted CBD to be used for CBD to treat medical conditions. These states were Wisconsin, Utah, Tennessee, South Carolina, North Carolina, Missouri, Mississippi, Kentucky, Iowa, Florida and Alabama. In various other countries, such as those of the United Kingdom, CBD has also been recognized as a legally-approved supplement.

The social, legal and political arenas are becoming less hostile in the usage of CBD oil for its therapeutic benefits A variety of techniques and services are available to make use of the healing properties of widely misunderstood and feared oil. There are many CBD water and lotions readily available that could have previously been unattainable in the past 30 years. CBD oil has been marketed for its ability to lower anxiety levels, relieve stress, reduce various types of aches and discomforts as well as reduce inflammation, reduce depression and can help reduce or even eliminate symptoms from ailments, pain as well as diseases. Certain individuals who are so enlightened in not relying on traditional painkillers, taking the decision to load their medical cabinets with jars and vials that contain CBD oil. If you suffer of mental illness, CBD oil has been proven to ease the issues. Athletes also frequently praise CBD oil's benefits. CBD oil. Typically, they rub the lotion on specific the areas of their body after an intense workout. Since CBD oil to have been in use for so long and had numerous benefits and uses demonstrated numerous times, it's impressive that the oil is able kept proving its authenticity. At least in some places there is a shift in the society aspects of their stance on hemp and marijuana. CBD oil is now allowed for doing the tasks that it excels at.

The reason why it has happened is due to the cannabinoids, which are the compounds that are found in cannabis sativa. They are the ones that give an array of medical and recreational characteristics of cannabis. There are more than 60 distinct cannabinoids that are unique to cannabis, and CDB is just one. The most famous of these cannabinoids is probably tetrahydrocannabinol, most often referred to simply as THC. THC is the compound which causes an alteration in consciousness (commonly called "being elevated") when you smoke, or other methods, to consume marijuana. The substance that alters your state of consciousness is referred to as a psychoactive substance. CBD is not psychoactive, or non-psychotropic substance, which means it doesn't alter a person's level of consciousness. It is not possible to get high CBD oil by using only CBD oil. Most, if not all varieties of marijuana contain greater amounts of THC than CBD. Getting CBD oil for use in therapeutic purposes was a challenge to conquer previously. Because CBD becomes more widely accepted and standardized, the extraction of just CBD with no THC has become more widespread and could remain so in the near future.

Legalizing marijuana is now the latest hot-button subject, with folks on both sides eager to provide a variety of theories and opinions in support of this, even when there was no demand for them to. The use of CBD oil to treat ailments is, however, been removed from the discussion about legalizing marijuana. It is likely that you live in a place where CBD oil is totally legally legal as well as safe from legal repercussions. If that's the case, it is your right to play to see whether it helps ease any medical issue that you may be suffering from, whether mental or physical, which is affecting you. The search for CBD oil isn't an issue also, since it's increasing in demand and ending onto more stores' shelves. If you are having trouble finding a shop that sells CBD oil, you can search online for a number of sites that provide it for sale and delivery. But, if you reside in a region where CBD oil is not yet frowned on, it needs been stated clearly that you shouldn't put yourself in a potentially harmful legal scenario. If this is the case, and it's unjust and unjust circumstances in your area and you are looking to find a more healthy and organic alternative to modern medical treatments apart from CBD oil. There are many types of brands selling CBD oil. As this is the case, consider taking time time following the guide to conduct the necessary research on your own and find out the details about the various brands that is available.

Be aware that this publication is not an alternative to your regular medical professional. Make sure to consult your physician before making any self-medications however it may be something that's as safe and dependable as CBD oil.

How Does CBD Oil Work?

The most commonly held belief concerning plants and herb (or in the case of this book an ingredient found inside the plants, specifically CBD oil) is that, when they are put into the body of a person it is when some gross or magical transformation occurs that can cause people to be better, more fit or more higher. Human brains don't necessarily work in this way. Though the process by which the brain functions is unsolved, it is being systematically decoded every as the years go by. Today's questions become the questions to the questions of the future.

There are various substances produced in the human body and are referred to as"endocannabinoids. In the human brain, there is a myriad of receptors that let us receive stimuli from outside and not allow any thing to be absorbed into our bodies however, they actually use whatever external stimuli might be. Imagine the antenna connected to your car, and consider comparing your brain with the your body. Consider the radio station that is located near that you are located. The radio station (external world) emits a signal (a music broadcast on radio) which is then received by your brain's diverse receptors (the antennas in the car). Without receptors inside our brains and body to receive all stimuli that comes from outside could just be a blur. Without these receptors, we'd not be in a position to taste, smell and hear, as well as feel and even be able to see or hear anything.

The Endocannabinoids receptors are located found in the brain and body that have been specifically programmed to us in order we are able to recognize and be aware of all diverse cannabinoids like THC or CBD which can be absorbed into the body's physiological system. The first receptor for cannabinoids wasn't discovered until 1998. Once it was confirmed to be present in our body scientists immediately began in search of an agonist for the receptor.

The term "ligand" can be described as a substance that is able to connect with receptors within our body. When a ligand is bound to any receptor it happens to be bound to, it may alter the way receptors work and behave. If THC connects to an receptor, it can frequently alter the behaviour and the structure of the receptor it is bonded to as well. Since THC has psychoactive properties, it brings to an alteration in the state of mind. That is, THC binds and acts as a ligand. It binds itself to receptors in the brain and alters the receptor to make it feel "high".

There is also CBD. Because CBD does not have psychoactive properties It will also be able to connect to receptors and, when it does so there is no sense of a elevated.

Concerning the endocannabinoid receptors two points that have to be uncovered. CB1 is the most important one that is located across different parts within the brain. The brain regions where they are the most abundant in include the motor aspects of the endocrinology system (automatic and manual control) and emotions, cognition, memory and sensory perception, as well as pain receptor, coordination as well as anything involving the movement.

The other endocannabinoid receptor you should pay attention to is CB2. They are located primarily within your immune system. As of now, science has established that they are responsible for the reduction of certain kinds of pains and aches, in addition to acting as a de-inflammatory.

It is becoming clear the fact that CBD is not any significant effect on CB1 as well as CB2 receptors. THC has a powerful influence on both CB1 as well as CB2 receptors. It is also psychoactive. This is for the reason that most cannabis that is used for recreational purposes has an enormous amount of CBD instead of THC. When you are using CBD oil, you'll benefit from the benefits of health which are present in the oil, but won't activate the areas of your brain which bring to an altered mental state.

In the process of extracting CBD of cannabis, it turns to a yellowish-looking oil. When it's turned into liquid, it could later add to water, or use in a similar way to different methods users make use of oils.

CBD Oil VS Hemp Oil

There are many different oils which can be made from Cannabis sativa plants. Marijuana oil THC oil cannabis oil CBD oil come from the same plant, however dependent on the way in which the plant is grown as well as the way in which the oil is extracted can determine the type of oils you can get as well as the purpose it could be utilized to use it for.

The majority of people talk about CBD oil, it could refer to it by the name of Hemp oil. That's not an untrue name in a scientific sense. It is not a good idea to group them in a single group, however. If you are referring to hemp oil must be known as hemp seed oil because it is more precise to the type of oil people are usually talking about.

The hemp seed oil has an attractive appearance. It is not like CBD oil. In the absence of knowing, you might have utilized hemp seed oil a number of times in the past. It's a popular ingredient in a variety of cosmetics as well as in some food items. The hemp seed oil is acknowledged to possess its own variety of positive effects and benefits. It is essential to make it absolutely explicit about the difference between hemp seed oil as well as CBD oil aren't exactly the same thing, even though they come from the identical plant. The amount of CBD within hemp seeds. For hemp seed oil, seeds are crushed into a liquid. CBD is derived from the plant but it is not from the seeds which will grow into plants if it is grown properly. There is a small amount of CBD which can be detected in the seeds, but not anywhere near enough to make a specific, useful, or useful use for the seeds. The hemp seed oil is not to be promoted or used as it has no medical or therapeutic benefits. The only place hemp seed oil's its best when it comes to the field of nutrition-perhaps the one area in which hemp seed oil is superior to CBD oil. In the case of extracting a chemical in the Cannabis sativa plant to use for reasons of health or therapeutic purposes, CBD oil trumps hemp seed oil by a wide margin.

CBD oil is not created from any variety of hemp. It's a particular breed that was bred specifically for particular purposes like producing topical applications, health advantages, and boosting fibre. The strains that are specifically bred for these purposes have a lower percentage of THC and significantly higher in CBD as compared to other varieties of hemp plant. Furthermore, when CBD extracts into an oil, it does by using whole plant, or the aerial portions. The aerial components are diverse areas within the plant that are continually and continuously exposed oxygen and air.

The most common way to extract CBD oil is to extract CBD oil from cannabis plant is by soaking the cannabis plant in carrier oil (typically olive oil) prior to doing any other thing. This helps to break down various components from the plant, and then extract what type of oil you're looking for which is in this instance CBD.

In the absence of THC there would not experience any psychoactive effects which are derived from the oil extracted from cannabis. The hemp seed oil nor the CBD oil contain THC If there is, then the amount would be small that they will not have any effect even on the youngest child, or for an adult who is fully grown.

In examining the holistic options to try to stay away from major pharmacy brands, CBD oil is one among the most frequently spoken about ingredients available. But it's important to be aware of the product you're making use of, and to not mix up one product with another. We should reiterate that hemp seed oil as well as CBD oil are distinct substances that are derived from the same source, and each has its own applications. If you're brand unfamiliar with the concept of CBD oil, making sure you aren't mixing one substance with the other is essential in making sure your knowledge is growing at a steady pace and speed.

The reason to use CBD Oil to start With?

Modern-day medical technology can be a frightening world to enter. The side effects can be numerous. In the office, waiting for hours, or for hours at a time will ruin every plan of not just one day, but could create chaos in the entire workweek of a person. Physicians, though essential and must be admired, may make a mistake or begin prescribing medications and pills for conditions that could only need the use of a gentle touch rather than an imposing hand with medication. Insurance companies have a tendency to boost rates and shock people who aren't aware of more changes to the medical plan and beliefs. The visit to the doctor may be more expensive than patients can afford. And there is no doubt of to see someone go into debt by simply visiting an office of a physician a couple times or one time. Some people prefer to skip treatment altogether and endure the pain and uncertainty due to the fact that going to a doctor or finding out how to cover the costs appears to be illogical, and unattainable.

Luckily, there are other options that are available, and CBD oil is only one. In the next chapters, we'll dive more deeply into exactly what CBD oil is able to be utilized to benefit. Once you're more familiar with the concept of CBD oil is, as well as what it's not as well, and you have a little more about the reasons it functions in the way it does, you'll enjoy all the health benefits CBD oil can provide.

In spite of the warnings previously given and the generally unnoticed negatives of seeing a physician It must be reiterated this guide isn't an attempt to replace your healthcare provider. Each medical treatment you engage in must be made by speaking with your physician.

Ask them any questions about CBD oil that you are interested in. They will also have information to impart about the topic. If you are asking questions to your doctor regarding CBD oil, they could be trying to divert you from the subject and also consider taking it in all. They may also be able to convince you otherwise. Doctors are exactly like everyone other. They share their faults as they have their merits. If a physician doesn't have a good understanding of CBD oil (or another topic) it is important to be aware that they might think that they've been in a tough spot.

Imagine being an educator in a class and you has a student asking questions about something that you are not familiar with yet you're expected to be a authority in. Human nature can take over, and the doctor could be embarrassment. They will then either shot off the notion completely and tell you that you have done something wrong by discussing something that is similar to CBD oil. They might even do something more sinister, such as making false stories, and exaggerating is true while telling you to take any CBD oil, all as they give your prescriptions for different medications. Naturally, there are doctors who, although probably not all of them, will be like that. However, humans are humans. There are some who behave in this manner even if you observe them in a bad day.

In fact, the opposite may occur. The doctor you see may have more information about CBD oil than any other person that you've ever spoken to before, however they may not intending to bring the subject up because of the debate surrounding its usage. Whatever the case, you're your own person to open the door about the subject and begin the conversation. Don't be shy and don't avoid bringing the topic of CBD oil with your doctor regardless of whether you don't agree with them but you must still conduct your own investigation.

Be sure to treat the health of your body seriously in all ways you are able to. At the end of the day, it is you to decide on your mind, body and overall wellbeing in every way.

Enjoy CBD Oil so far? Send your thoughts with the entire world!

Chapter 2: Types Of Cbd Oil

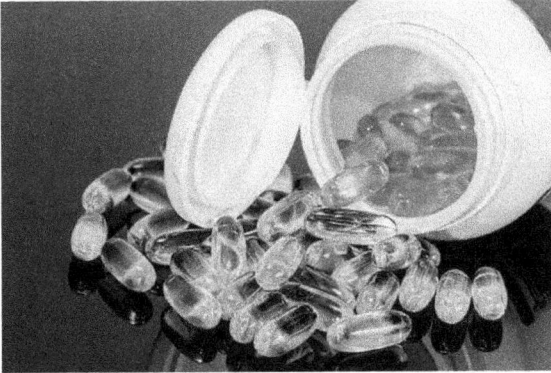

The health benefits of using CBD oil are numerous and numerous. Contrary to traditional medications that have precise sometimes unclear and unpractical directions to administer them, oil that are used to treat ailments tend to be with a lot less hassle, and they can even be enjoyable to use. In general, CBD oil extracts are consumed by way of tablets or gels, and sometimes an oral pill.

There are many other strategies to make use of CBD oil, however we'll go over these for you in order to improve your understanding and the usage of CBD oil simpler. Like we said earlier the use of CBD oil is not going to cause any kind of a buzz however it can cause you to feel good, at ease, relaxed and create a feeling of calm.

The term used to describe the method that uses CBD oil is usually called cannabidiol delivery. There are generally four options for this type of delivery. Each of these is safe and simple to comprehend While one has a distinct taste. However, every method must be thoroughly explained to ensure you know the implications of each.

Be assured As you continue studying, I'm certain you'll realize that you don't have anything to worry about as the negative effects associated with CBD oil are virtually non-existent However, the more you are aware of, the better you'll feel. The more you know, the better you hear, and shifting away from contemporary medical practice to something that is more holistic, building your own power is exactly what this article is about.

The Different Methods of Using CBD Oil Medicinally and Therapeutically

Be aware about the health issue you are suffering from prior to applying any of these techniques. In certain situations, one method of making use of CBD oil could be more effective than the other. Whatever condition you're facing take the time to test a variety of ways to determine which is the most effective for your needs.

If there's any kids or teens who have read this book Be sure to check with your parents before utilizing CBD oil or other natural substance that is intended to treat medical conditions or for any other purpose.

Inhalation

The initial method of delivery is to inhale the oil. It is only recommended by those who are adults and have past history of vaping including vape pens used to substitute or duplicate cigarettes and vaporizers that are standard (the ones used to inhale vapors of citrus and other fruit) or any other device related to this. If you already are smoker, it is an easy and pleasant method to introduce the CBD oil into your body. If you don't have experience with vaping it is possible to explore alternative options described below. If you are not a smoker, the task of figuring out how to breathe rightly will be viewed more like a hassle more than any other. Avoid the additional hassle and focus on alternatives. To be clear Inhaling CBD (or any that isn't the fumes) generally means you're inhaling CBD. It is important not to make your dreams come true or sabotage any other thoughts you have- CBD oil doesn't contain THC, and won't give you a high even if you do smoke it.

Inhaling CBD oil might be the most powerful and effective method of reaping the advantages. Inhaling CBD oil can provide you with much more of the authentic and purest CBD oil than you would with other approaches. Inhaling cannabidiol does not only enter your lung, but it will also enter it will also enter the bloodstream. There are many benefits of CBD oil, bloodstream is the place you would like the oil to move. Anything that cannabidiol-containing product enters the body via this route will quickly be absorbed into bloodstream and bypass liver. Additionally, any hemp products inhaled (next to TCH and marijuana) generally leave the bloodstream in just several hours. But, it is possible that different results occur for various people.

There's a huge selection of CBD oils available which are readily available to purchase. The process of analyzing each one of them is an overwhelming undertaking, therefore it is necessary to test several different kinds and find what you prefer. There's a flavour for everyone. If you're someone who is already vaping the best thing to do is take this route for a start to the vast ocean of CBD oil. If smoking CBD oil is how you go about it this means that you will not just be receiving all the health benefits and benefits, but you can even discover a new pastime or simply the extension of an existing one if you've already been vaping.

If you are a parent that are reading this, there's one thing I would like you to remember. Inhaling CBD oil via vapes is like smoking tobacco or inhaling tobacco, and letting your kids access their CBD oil via vaping could be a way to teach them some behaviors that should not be allowed to develop later on with different things other than CBD. If you're an adult and taking in CBD is your method of choice to incorporate CBD in your body, it needs been suggested not to let your children do the same as you do, or be able to use a vape before the kids. Naturally, this is an individual choice, and there is no rights to dictate the best way to raise their children. However, it is still necessary to be clarified in the end.

Sublingual

Sublingual refers to "under the tongue". This technique is employed to create CBD extracts, which are available as concentrations and tinctures. They typically refer to the pure CBD oil. Therefore, you will get results that are quick to take effect. After placing CBD oil on your tongue, capillaries within the mucous membranes are able to take it in and then send it into the bloodstream. After that, the remainder of the substance you put on your tongue is safe to swallow. The oil is safe to digest, and it should not cause any discomfort. The people who have utilized this method to get CBD oil into their bodies frequently report that the results appear quick, sometimes even immediately and last for an extended time.

Instructions for using sublingual methods are incredibly simple. If you are a parent who are out there, this could be an effective option to help get CBD oil in your child with no range of headaches and complaints. The only thing you have to do is put the CBD in the mouth and leave it there for at least a minute half, up to 2 minutes. After 2 minutes it is believed that the CBD will be absorbed through the mucous membranes. In this method it is likely that both the liver and digestive system will be eliminated, and the CBD goes straight to the bloodstream, however the tincture containing CBT won't remain in the bloodstream, but it will be consumed and consumed. Once CBD oil is consumed, CBD oil gets into the bloodstream through this process, it'll make it's way into the endocannabinoid organs very swiftly.

Topical Application

This is a well-known one which also helps to soothe the skin. It also causes it feeling relaxed in the beginning, before CBD starts to work. While certain CBD application on the skin provide type of gentle and calming sensation, but there are many readily available and also function as cosmetic and skincare items. Because CBD oil is growing in the market, more advantages have been discovered and the shift from CBD topically applied oil used to boost health and wellness to the world of skin and beauty was an easy decision.

The other benefit of making use of CBD oil in this manner is the fact that it gets straight into the targeted region in the human body. This is because, when you apply CBD oil on the skin is usually as a cream or lotion. It is an effective and popular method to reduce the discomfort caused by the inflammation of joints, stiffness and other types of pain to hands and other areas where it needs to be addressed. Additionally, it can help alleviate muscles that are stressed or decrease irritations to the skin, such as rashes. As you can see, there's some connection with the beauty industry and skincare, there's plenty of scents and fragrances to enjoy with CBD oil application.

There are so many kinds of CBD creams and lotions as the variety of flavours for vaping. This is another illustration of the ways in which CBD is able to be utilized for much more than what it was meant to be. The benefits of this wonderful oil are certainly infinite in their possibilities. There's even been a story that has been circulating online and a small viral product that you might have heard about that is known as CBD bath bomb. CBD bath bomb.

Consuming the oil in the form of a tablet, spray with water or mixed with food.

This is the simplest and most beginner approach to obtain a dose CBD oil. If you are just beginning and with no desire to try alternative methods such as kids or for those that prefer to take their CBD oil in a short time, similar to using a typical everyday pills it is the ideal method to take. Simply take a tablet-like one or two tabs and put the tablets into your mouth. Then drink it in an ice cube and you're done with the CBD oil analysis throughout your entire daily. Pills are able to concentrate what's inside of them, which is the reason they're the most common method to distribute a range of drugs in the field of health. The vitamins we consume each day function in the similar way, and CBD oil supplements aren't any different.

There is no instruction or education required to obtain CBD oil into your system. If you take CBD oil as a pill the pill will go through the digestive system prior to it reaches the liver. When it reaches the liver, it'll begin to process. It is then that the concentration of CBD oil is released through the bloodstream. CBD oil pills are used just like every other type of supplement with no concern about side effects or a strange backlash. Most people should be able to take pills with no difficulty or effort.

A different method of administration that is popular and doesn't require any formal instruction is to get your daily dose of CBD by spray. The process is similar to other types of medical sprays. Simply spray a small amount into your mouth, and it will behave as if it were pills. This is another option that is used by those with little knowledge or are reluctant to try different methods. It is an easy way to keep track of the amount of CBD oil consumption.

There are a variety of ways of how CBD oil is directly taken in. One of the simplest and popular ways is mixing the CBD oil and water. They can be purchased in a retail store, or you could mix the oil and the water by yourself. Any way works. This approach is ideal for those who are constantly moving and don't have the time to relax. If you decide to mix CBD oil with water you drink on your own the only thing you need to do is ensure you've got the dosage correct and ensure that you consume all the water you drink throughout the day. That's it! You can then transport it anywhere and sip at your convenience without worrying about breaking any of it down into a schedule. This is also a common way to consume CBD oil by athletes, who tend to approach CBD oil just as you would treat a bottle Gatorade or other electrolyte product. If your daily life is moving and you're constantly traveling from one spot to the next, then you must begin using CBD oil by this method.

A spray or pill isn't the only option to consume CBD oil, however. It is also able to be added to food items and eaten through eating. It's dependent on you whether you decide to take in this direction with CBD oil. However, it's something that you should test at least once. Perhaps you'll find a flavorful topping you can use to your favourite recipes. Some of the most inventive individuals are coming up with many different methods to include CBD oil into food. If you've been wanting to test this out We have couple of ideas to bring your mind to the brink.

Combine CBD oil with pesto, and make pizza.

Mix some CBD oil into a smoothie of fruit and enjoy the refreshing drink of health! For a boost in the health benefits of your drink, prepare the smoothie using wheatgrass.

Mix some CBD oil and chocolate to enjoy your palate with some pleasure. Truffles are great when paired when paired with CBD oil.

Beer. Yes, even though you know that CBD oil isn't a source of THC, you'll still be able to enjoy a bit of a blast while enjoying the benefits for health from the oil. Cannabis and hops are closely related, and the notion to keep it within the same family as nature's other animals is not a big leap.

Add a little CBD oil into your cup of coffee before you get going.

The next time you are sitting at a table to watch a film then why not swap off the butter and opt for CBD oil?

When you cook any kind of recipes that require olive oil include a drop of CBD oil to your recipe. A lot of chefs and cooks have made it a regular practice, and it's popularity is likely to keep growing.

You can also find other candy and gummies available sold on the market, which contain CBD in them.

How Do You Want Your Oil?

As you can see, there is a variety of ways to make use of CBD oil. These methods all serve various objectives and when the use of CBD oil for physical, mental and physical ailments, selecting the correct technique is essential. The immediate introduction of CBD oil to your body, similar to tablets and foods will be the optimally. Applying CBD oil on your tongue can also work like the consumption of it. In order to calm the nerves, and putting the brain in more positive state applying topical ointments or taking it inhalation can work. Making sure you use it in the right way is dependent to the kind of issue you're trying to eliminate. If you are suffering from multiple issues, then mixing a few strategies will assist you in finding a healthier general health.

Chapter 3: Using Cbd Oil Against Illness

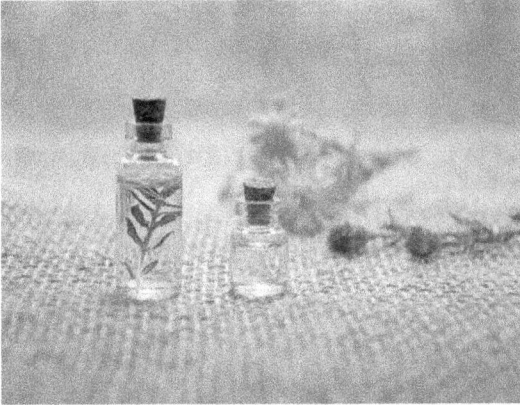

Now that you have some basic information about the basics of what CBD is and how it functions as well as the various methods you can use to benefit from it, you are now able using CBD oil to do its best use. There are many different conflicts and diseases which CBD oil may help reduce.

If you are using CBD oil for purposes for health, it's important to understand the results you're looking for. The term "illness" is a broad term and sometimes ambiguous.

There are three types of ailments that a person might be battling. It could be mental, physical or diseases. The term "pain" is used to describe the symptoms of physical disease. Stress, anxiety as well as neurological issues fall under the umbrella of mental illnesses. In addition, most of the most common illnesses that patients justifiably worry about and aren't willing to discuss for too long time, are classified under general health and wellness.

A diagnosis of a condition can be a difficult thing to deal with. The general condition is a burden on mental and physical health, and is often the effect of bringing down negativity that affects not only the person that has been afflicted as having a condition and on other individuals around them too. The use of CBD oil isn't an enchantment. It's not a magical remedy that can cure illnesses and all of issues in life just by taking it on a regular basis or once. It should be utilized alongside the required adjustments to lifestyle, guidelines given by a medical professional as well as any other medication or procedure is needed to combat any illness.

Don't be swayed and believe that the medical field is a bad thing. Herbal remedies and holistic herbs are appearing on the scene and the medical profession, having lots of money involved just isn't a rebel against a competitor who is trying to eat a slice from the cake. There's no reason for us to believe that standard treatments for medical conditions shouldn't be paired with CBD oil, or other treatment that is natural.

If more holistic solutions have been proven to be effective and widely accepted by the medical profession, they is expected to integrate these into their routine practices. The bigwigs and suitors who decide on patients' healthcare do not fall aligned with CBD oil or holistic therapies However, medical professionals and nurses who do their real-world fieldwork and provide treatment for those who need it have chosen their careers using the highest of motives and are to be trusted. Ask them questions about CBD oil. They're the ones who have the closest relationship with you, and who understand what's going on regarding your health. by combining the latest medical information combined with natural treatments You will get all the benefits available from both side of the spectrum.

These ailments that CBD Oil Treats can be used to fight

Because CBD oil, while not a new discovery, it is increasing in therapeutic purposes, there are a few regions that are backed by a wealth of data that is solid, whereas other areas aren't. In spite of this disparity across the board, CBD oil has already been proven to aid in fighting against a variety of health problems.

In some cases, CBD oil is able to directly defend against issues, while for other conditions, it can just reduce the symptoms. These two, good and the bad, features and benefits of CBD oil may be a little bit more importance when looking for ways to improve general well-being. If you're looking to become more healthy, each little step will make a difference.

Cancer

One of the most prominent names that come on the screen when people start to take CBD oil is that of cancer. While research is still in its early stages of finding out the ways in which CBD helps fight cancer, outcomes are promising thus far. In the meantime, National Cancer Institute has leapt into the challenge of trying to discover the effectiveness of CBD oil is in warding against cancer. The institute isn't yet ready to support CBD oil or any product connected to cannabis for stopping or preventing the growth of cancer cells. However, they haven't shied away from any positive evidence that has emerged. There is evidence that CBD oil is anti-inflammatory, and also alter the way specific cells reproduce. Tumor cells can be included in this. Initial reports point towards the possibility that CBD oil could decrease the size of certain cancer cells, as well as the ability to stop them from reproducing completely.

The breast cancer issue has been recognized and proved that it is the most promising in the field of CBD oil. An investigation conducted in 2006 demonstrated for the very first time that CBD oil can block different kinds of breast tumor cells. The effects were powerful and can't be ignored or overlooked. Tested on cells that were not cancerous they showed effects that were lower in intensity, which led to the realization that CBD oil is a direct weapon against cancer cells in a specific way. CBD oil is believed to have both anti-proliferative and pro-apoptotic impacts that may cause tumor cell proliferation to block its invasion, adhesion and.

A different research study was conducted in the year 2011 provided the world with a more comprehensive understanding of the data they could utilize. Researchers found that CBD oil could cause the death of breast cancer cells, without affecting the surrounding tissue. The death of a concentrated and dependent group of cells that are located in two receptors (estrogen receptor positive and estrogen receptor negative) has been observed to happen after CBD oil was introduced into cells. As the amounts of CBD did not have any influence on the mammary cell and the other cells that are not tumor-causing which is great news. It was evident the effectiveness of using CBD to fight breast cancer, and other regions of the body without signs of tumors or other symptoms were not affected by negative side negative effects. A separate study found that for patients suffering from discomfort related to cancer, and were not receiving relief from any other medications treatment options, CBD oil could provide significant relief.

Additionally, there has been evidence collected that have given evidence in the use of CBD oil for overcoming not just cancer in its entirety, but also to help alleviate signs and symptoms associated with cancer and side consequences of chemotherapy. One of the most significant negative side effects associated with chemotherapy are nausea and vomiting. These are both reduced when using CBD oil.

The dosage currently recommended to use CBD for fighting cancer is 700 mg taken every day for six weeks. There was no evidence of toxicity in this dose, which leads some to believe CBD oil is a viable option in conjunction with an ongoing treatment program.

While the majority of tests which have been conducted regarding CBD oil as well as cancer were conducted in lab animals and more data from humans must be collected before taking any fact as a matter of fact however, breast cancer isn't the only type of cancer that could be susceptible in CBD oil. Colon lung cancer, colon and leukemia might also be less difficult to conquer when you incorporate CBD in a plan of treatment. As CBD is accepted as a treatment and accepted, the clinical data required continues to arrive.

Diabetes

It's been demonstrated that CBD has the ability to reduce the risk that mice develop diabetes. up to 56 percent the reduction in inflammation was achieved. In addition to research involving mice, it's been demonstrated that CBD may reduce the levels in plasma of proinflammatory Cytokines.

Certain studies have been carried out also on human subjects. Particularly, one 2013 was conducted to determine what link or connection existed between the use of marijuana and insulin the resistance to insulin, and glucose. There were 4,657 individuals took part in the experiment between 2005 and 2010. One-third of those who participated were previous marijuana users, and 579 still taking the drug during the time of the research. At the conclusion of the research the results showed that those who used marijuana for a long time had a reduction of 16 percent in levels of insulin all over the board. Also, it was observed that people who had been taking marijuana exhibited a slimmer waistline. It wasn't something could be believed to be true, however having a greater circumference around your waist could cause the onset of diabetes. As with cancer and as time progresses there will be more testing by humans, as well as hard evidence will be released for helping to connect the dots of CBD oil and the treatment of the effects of diabetes.

Heart Health

There is a direct connection established between CBD oil and lower blood pressure. An experiment of a small size was carried out using 10 male participants. The participants were given only one dose of 600 milligrams CBD oil. Each of them experienced reduced blood pressure after taking CBD oil. CBD oil. Researchers who conducted the study further probed more deeply. The male subjects received stress tests which generally result in high blood pressure when they're done. They discovered that a single dose consumed of CBD oil helped them through these tests. At the conclusion of the tests, subjects showed only a small rise in blood pressure, in comparison to the usual pace of growth.

A lower blood pressure beneficial for all of the cardiovascular system. That also includes heart. If blood pressures are reduced, so too are the risk of having heart attacks, metabolic syndrome as well as having a stroke. There is also another less well-known disease called vascular hyperpermeability (which may result in leaky stomach) which has seen to be lowered with CBD oil. CBD oil also helps remove any excess cholesterol may have been accumulating in the body of a person.

Through tests on animals, CBD oil has shown similar results in relation to general cardiovascular well-being. Cell death and the death of cells associated with heart disease as well as inflammations have been proven to decrease when mice have been treated with CBD oil supplied to the mice. CBD oil has also been proven to decrease oxidative stress and can even stop damage to the heart from extending further in mice.

Acne

While acne isn't more serious than those in this section however, it's an issue that many people struggle with. The problem isn't just limited to teens also. A lot of adults struggle dealing with acne issues on regular every day basis. Fortunately, CBD oil could help you with this as well.

There are a variety of causes that trigger acne to show its unattractive face. Genetics and bacteria are two of the most popular causes. However, acne may cause inflammations as well. It is said that CBD oil can be a powerful anti-inflammatory, and can assist reduce the amount of cells that are causing the acne condition to develop.

A third major reason for acne can be attributed to something known as sebum. If the body produces more sebum than is required, there may result in a physiological reaction which causes glands to release oily substances throughout the face. This is a problem that can be addressed through the use of CBD oil. CBD may help to reduce and stop the production of sebum and reduce the appearance of acne.

Other Diseases

The ailments listed in this section are ones in which hard data have already been collected. While more information remains needed to discover more about the advantages of the use of CBD oil for treatment, the avenue of understanding has started to become clearer and additional time will be required. There are many other medical issues which CBD is proven to be able to solve. There are many other.

CBD oil has been found to boost appetite.

Reduced inflammation in digestive diseases like ulcerative colitis and Crohn's disease.

Chapter 4: Using Cbd Oil To Curb Pain

Atural pain relief is the thing that can put CBD oil right in the spotlight. Of the numerous advocates that advocate the usage of CBD oil, relieving discomfort is the most prominent reason and argument they use. It shouldn't be any unexpected shock. Marijuana generally is used for reducing the pain for a long time before doctors has ever prescribed the first prescription for a medically-approved pill. Utilizing marijuana to ease pain is documented from as early as 2900 BC. Even though THC is likely to play a role in this, at a minimum extent, the main reasons marijuana has the capability of relieving pain is due to the fact that it is a transporter in CBD oil.

Do you remember the endocannabinoids discussed earlier? These substances do more than simply determine what molecules are connected to receptors in the nervous system. They are also involved in controlling the activity of your immune system, making it easier to induce sleep and regulating the rate of appetite and detecting or lessening the discomfort. Once the receptors for endocannabinoids start to activate and causing pain, they should decrease. It is possible to sense there's a pain somewhere within the body, and then go into action, making painful sensation less obvious.

An experiment conducted on rats was able to confirm the point further. The animals were given small surgical cuts. They then received an amount of CBD oil. The rodents showed less of the pain sensation and, instead of drowning in the pain, they returned to normal behaviors more quickly than the normal. Another study conducted with rats related to inflammation and the sciatic nerve. The rats received oral CBD oil treatment. Like the animals who were treated with surgical cuts those who were given the oral CBD oil doses recovered to their normal behaviour faster than they might have had been otherwise.

When it comes to studies for humans are concerned, small number of these are being conducted. The majority of them were conducted to determine what advantages CBD oil can provide sufferers of discomfort from rheumatoid arthritis as well as MS. A number of countries across the globe have cleared CBD oil to reduce discomfort for those suffering from these conditions.

As more than 40 individuals (who were all diagnosed with MS) were brought together for the purpose of a study and all were provided with a dose of CBD oil via the use of an orally sprayed. The test ran for the entire month. Results came back exactly as the participants wanted them to. Participants in the study claimed to have felt an improvement in pain when compared with other participants who were provided with different placebos as opposed to CBD oil. The specific areas of pain examined for the research were muscle spasms, and problems getting around. To all those who are struggling with MS You should know there are others who claimed that CBD oil has allowed their ability to walk and lead a life with a bit more ease. Some countries are already ahead of the CBD medical revolution by permitting CBD oil utilized as a treatment for pain caused from multiple sclerosis. In these countries, Canada and the United Kingdom are the leaders in the global game, and are waiting for the remaining nations of the world to get on the same page. There is still a disagreements going on about this subject. There is no way to know whether CBD oil as a sole agent to relieve the pain that is a result of MS. A lot of CBD delivery methods that Canada as well as in the United Kingdom use also contain THC.

It could be primarily CBD oil which helps lessen chronic pain, but the THC might also play part in the process. In any case, CBD oil has been proven to be effective in more than one instance to alleviate the pain and suffering associated with MS. It could be the day that the various cultures around all over the world come together to find the root of what benefits from CBD oil from the Cannabis sativa plant is, rather than tearing everything into pieces and creating more confusion and arguments, however currently in the majority of countries, CBD oil as well as THC need to be purchased independently. If the region you reside within has a negative opinion about THC or is illegal in its entirety however, you'll have the ability to get some comfort by using only plain and unadulterated CBD oil.

The National Institutes of Health have taken the initiative to find out some more details on CBD oil. They have taken a look at the possibilities possible ways to reduce pain after using chemotherapy. The reason the reason for using chemotherapy initially. Chemotherapy helps fight to eliminate, kill, or destroy cancerous cells. There's no better reason to take chemotherapy. As devastating as it is to mention, chemotherapy could be extremely stressful on a patient through. The treatment is not only effective in fighting cancer, but also causes tremendous pain for patients throughout their recuperation process. It is good news that CBD oil has demonstrated an upside of the pain-inducing side effects of chemotherapy. According to reports, those who've undergone chemotherapy say they experienced a reduction in pain following the use of CBD oil. Due to this, the addition of CBD oil usage in conjunction chemotherapy has become an increasingly common practice.

If you've been diagnosed with rheumatoid arthritis the same results have been verified. According to reports, those who suffer from the condition on a daily day basis, they've mentioned being more comfortable when they take a dosage of

CBD oil. In addition, it has been found to lessen stiffness and pain caused by arthritis, but a lot of people affected by the disease claim that CBD oil can help them to sleep more peacefully during the evening. This isn't just restricted for those who are unable to sleep due to arthritis. anyone who struggles to get an adequate night's sleep could also benefit from CBD oil to help with this.

The condition of insomnia is among the most prevalent medical conditions that humanity has ever faced. About a third of all people in any time throughout history, have difficulties sleeping during the night as a result of sleeplessness. Inability to get the right sleep and insomnia can be the cause of pain. However, each and every cell of the body functions as an intricate web. When one region is afflicted by something, there can be a chain reaction that can cause problems within the body. Although a lack of sleep isn't directly causing discomfort, it is certainly not making anyone better off than in the event of getting adequate sleep. In addition, if there's an absence of sleep and the immune system can become disoriented and may not function properly. And, even more importantly, during sleep it is when the cells in the human body recover in a more effective pace. When you don't get adequate sleep and rest, any discomfort or discomfort you are suffering due to will take a longer time to be healed and get it fixed. Another reason to include CBD oil in your cupboard and quit using medications that are prescribed excessively quickly and often in excess. If you're getting more and longer sleep You will experience less discomfort overall. CBD oil might be what you require to get a trip into the dream.

In some instances, CBD oil has become an item that people who don't want to spend a second on anything depend on. Doctors, surgeons, paramedics and a myriad of roles in the medical sector are often in scenarios that can be literally life or death to a patient. Emergency situations can happen even if everyone would prefer they didn't. If you are when they are in emergency situations it's not enough time to consider, think about or estimate and then hope that it all happens. In the event that someone requires emergency medical treatment immediately, it is imperative to provide pain relief promptly and quickly. Together with morphine, as well as other fast-acting drugs CBD oil is added to the list essential medicines utilized in the most dire situations and scenarios.

In addition to multiple sclerosis as well as the negative effects being treated with chemotherapy Rheumatoid arthritis and urgent pain relief, there's different areas in which CBD oil is studying for the purpose of reducing chronic discomfort. Pain and general muscle aches caused by the spinal cord could be the next dark era that CBD oil will bring vital sunshine. As CBD oil is proving it's worth more and more it will be a subject of research that will keep on coming in, and we'll certainly find ways to resolve one of the longest-running and painful issues.

Apart from the most severe or debilitating pains which were mentioned CBD oil may also be employed to alleviate minor pains and inflammations. Topical ointments, applications and ointments described in the chapter 2 are brought into the picture here. As a result of living a regular lifestyle all day long and out, a person will begin feeling various ailments. This can occur due to performing sports, stretching incorrectly and gaining weight. It can also happen due to getting older, or with no cause at all. If one of these happens to you, it is possible to rub CBD oil over the region that is affected and you will begin feeling relief in a matter of minutes.

Another well-known illustration of CBD oil used for pain relief and show immediate results has been reported by an unknowing source. MMA boxer Nate Diaz is an avid user of CBD oil. It's not hard to believe that an elite fighter is lacking expertise in how to deal with and manage the pain. There is no way I can be an MMA professional, but when someone talks about the best ways to deal with many different pains I'll be listening. Nate Diaz can regularly be found smoking CBD oil, and has did it after the fight had ended after the match, while the press conference was going in.

Although some have criticized him because he promotes CBD oil in such a large amount and in such a way If someone fighting on a daily basis is making use of it to combat the pain of their body, it is bound worked pretty well. Additionally, nobody can say Nate Diaz is out of good shape or in poor well-being.

Chapter 5: Using Cbd Oil For Mental Health And Anxiety

A While it is gruelling to live with physical debilitating ailments and pain is, psychological pain can be equally difficult and, in some cases, more challenging to live in. Keep in mind that there's an unbeatable trifecta in relation to ailments that are medical. There's physical suffering, illness and mental wellness. There are a lot of those who wake each and every day to struggle through a life in which their mental health is not functioning fully, CBD oil is there to help them too.

Epilepsy

Epilepsy was the first condition in medicine which CBD oil has been proven to be effective in combating. Epilepsy is a condition that affects people with epilepsy. they're at risk of having seizures. Additionally, there are certain parts of their brain which are prone to the phenomenon of excitability. This is due to the fact that cannabinoids after being absorbed into the bloodstream, bind to those brain cells which manage the region of excitation that could trigger seizures. In this way, the amount of the excitability of the brain is controlled and managed enough to stop seizures from occurring again. In this area, there is a need for more solid data. In medical research there's never an issue as having sufficient information. The more details are on fingertips, the better can be for everybody. However, even experts from the American Epileptic Society has jumped into the fray in an effort to comprehend the ways in which CBD oil may be used to alleviate the signs as well as seizures associated with epilepsy.

A study was conducted in the year 2016 that included more than 200 participants who were all suffering from epilepsy. Participants were provided with doses taken by mouth of CBD oil each day. The doses varied from 2 to 5 milligrams. Over the course of 12 weeks, subjects were assessed for signs of any adverse side effects and also had the frequency of their seizures documented. In the case of more than 70 percent of them the seizures decreased to around 40 percent.

A different study was conducted in collaboration with Stanford University. This research specifically sought out on the internet parents of epilepsy children to come ahead. The reason to find individuals who would be interested in determining if CBD oil can provide any benefit for those with epilepsy. 19 volunteers were identified before the testing began to be conducted. The number of medications used in treating epilepsy among the people who were taking part in the test was estimated to be twelve. Although it was determined that people were more alert as well as having an improvement in mood were observed however, the most pleasing aspect for everyone involved was the reduction in epileptic issues that were noted. Six volunteers reported that they experienced a decrease of seizures between 25 and 60 percent reduction. Eight of the participants reported an increase of seizures that were reduced by around 80 percent. The most shocking part is that two patients reported that their seizures stopped entirely!

Anxiety and Depression

It is one of the areas where there's practically no discussion. CBD oil can help reduce anxiety and is extremely effective. If you are suffering with anxiety related to social interactions, CBD oil will help in overcoming it. The other types of anxiety being studied using CBD oil include anxiety disorder and post-traumatic stress disorder (PTSD) depression, obsessive-compulsive disorder and many more.

CBD oil releases dopamine in your body. In this way, feelings of joy will occur. CBD oil has also been proven to ease various tensions. If you do not suffer from any specific medical issue and you are not suffering from any particular illness, CBD oil is still able to be utilized during a hectic day, to get away from the stress and relax. It is not just that CBD oil help release dopamine but it may also change the manner in which your brain's receptors communicate with serotonin. Serotonin is a substance that has a direct connection to all parts of the mental well-being. In the end, the moment serotonin flows freely and is not being inhibited in a way that is incorrect then you can let the stress water roll over your shoulders.

An investigation conducted in 2011 was focused on public speaking and those with a Social anxiety disorder. 24 people with this disorder were chosen. Certain of them were treated with CBD oil, while the others received different alternative drugs. The experiment was conducted approximately an hour and half prior to the students being asked to speak in public. Results were exactly as expected. The people who did not receive CBD oil, they showed a greater degree of discomfort, anxiety and cognitive impairment. When they were provided with CBD oil demonstrated increased focus and enthusiasm when making speeches, which suggested that CBD oil was able to help calm the nerves and help them focus in the present.

The most significant and persistent issue which is encountered when treating any kind of depression or anxiety is the drugs employed to treat depression or anxiety. The medications are given with good intentions but the adverse effects associated with them could result in the opposite of what these great intentions intend to achieve. For starters, a lot of antidepressants may become addictive. And once someone decides to stop having them, they'll rapidly realize they aren't able to stop reaching for the bottle. And then, the depression could be back, and at the end, it is clear that the person had completed a complete cycle and is back exactly at the point they started at the beginning. This can create an unsettling pattern, but once they stop taking the medication, they might fall into a more depressed state as the one they began in at the beginning.

While CBD oil may help beat the mental illness of depression, there's no real cure for depression, other than one thing which is that a patient must over come a trauma or an event that changed the way they think about themselves and pushed to a depressive state in the first place. This is among the most difficult challenges every person will encounter, and a lot of people do not have the determination to persevere all the way to the finish. To no more feel down the need to modify the way the brain functions. The brain must be able to produce more positive chemicals produced in their brains, which can lead to higher levels of positive emotion.

It is not my intention to go more detail on how complicated process works as that's not the purpose in this guide. It should however be clear although CBD oil is a great way to reduce stress levels and stabilize you however, depression of any kind which someone might be suffering through must not be managed only by the person who is suffering. Seek out a professional or therapist of some kind. If the cost for therapy is excessive and is not in your budget real-world situation, consult a close friend or family member.

If it isn't feasible to do so you can read books on the subject or talk to someone on the internet or read others' stories to see what they did to change their mental model to become more positive. You can change your way of life or do something other than fighting the struggle on your own. CBD oil is a great way to combat depression. But to fully overcome it, you'll be required to alter something else regarding your lifestyle in addition. You can do itso don't think about it again.

But, as CBD oil is found to ease tension in muscles and nerves and reduce tension, it can help you relax that can allow you to letting depression go. CBD oil also helps people get more sleep and help in aiding people to get into a more positive mood.

If you've been diagnosed as having PTSD The use of CBD oil along with getting help from psychiatrists can help reduce anxiety and ease tension.

Stroke

A stroke is among the most terrifying experiences that a single person will ever endure. However, CBD oil has been proven the ability to assist those who are unfortunate enough of experiencing this. CBD is able to reduce in size the region of the brain where was attacked by the stroke!

In this way, CBD oil acts as a an insulator and help protect the brain from becoming worse following an accident. Similar studies in CBD oil are also associated with concussions.

Neurological Disorders

CBD oil can reduce the development and spread of Alzheimer's disease. While many aspects about Alzheimer's disease are still a mystery however, we know that amyloid plaques may be related to the disease. The active compounds in cannabis oil will stop amyloid plaques from forming.

CBD oil has also demonstrated potential in removing those who are addicted to drugs. Through a neurological process called neuroplasticity CBD oil has the ability to rewire brains and in the process it can help to replace the neural circuitry which has led addiction to an opioid drug. The tests have been conducted with animals to date However, the rats evaluated showed less dependence to heroin or Morphine after receiving the dose of CBD oil.

Keep in mind to keep in mind that CBD oil has a powerful anti-inflammatory. As it is, may help in many neurological conditions.

If you're affected by Parkinson's disease CBD oil has been proven that it can aid in to more sleep. In addition, a handful of patients suffering from Parkinson's disease claimed that CBD oil could help lessen pain, they've added that it may help reduce sleep shaking. Other people have reported that motor functions could improve overall. But, Parkinson's disease is among the grey zones in CBD oil usage. Even though CBD oil is not well-known as having an abundance of negative side effects while some individuals suffering from Parkinson's disease claimed that CBD oil has assisted those suffering with the condition have said exactly the opposite. There are a few instances where those suffering from Parkinson's disease reported that following the use of CBD oil the spasms, muscle movement, and night shaking only increased. Further research is required in relation to CBD oil and Parkinson's disease prior to gaining full certainty for recommending CBD oil can be granted.

Antipsychotic

It is essential to collect more data regarding how efficient CBD oil could be in combating the symptoms of mania. Schizophrenia is often featured on this site. According to some reports it is believed that the pharmacological profile of CBD oil may be described as being quite similar to the other antipsychotic drugs that are atypical. Like many studies that have been conducted in the past, they have mostly been conducted on animals. However, they do provide belief that CBD oil could in the future be the solution to putting someone who has mental illness onto a path towards better well-being.

It is similar to depression. Don't believe that CBD oil can cure any mental condition you suffer from. You should seek assistance from a professional if you're experiencing a misinterpretation of the world. This can certainly help, but figuring out the cause of the problem and moving to resolve it is the best method to identify the pieces that make up an a bit fractured mind prior to they can be put to its original form. I am not going to preach a falsehood and claim I know what it's like to live with any kind of mental illness can be like. I do never insult the intelligence of anyone with my flims assertion. Begin by taking CBD oil. CBD oil. However, you should also look for other assistance if you believe you require assistance. Always have someone you can go to when you really need assistance in any way.

Chapter 6: Cbd Oil Roundup

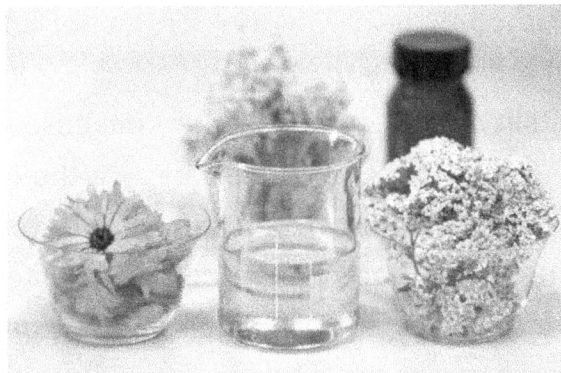

Thank you for coming to this point. It's not just a common complain, but an authentic gesture of thanks. In the case of any type of medical or physical condition doing the most basic of tasks such as the reading of a book is not a tiny feat for people who are able to accomplish it. You can be proud of yourself because there's nothing that is an unimportant accomplishment.

In the beginning, when you first enter the realm of CBD oil, the possibilities and details may seem a little overwhelming. It is likely that you will seen that there's really not too much to worry about. The adverse effects associated with CBD oil are very minor and, often it is unlikely to be observed. There is a possibility of experiencing an increase in appetite or you might feel sleepy although there are more important things to do than getting a bit more hungry and exhausted. The other side effects common to people who have been observed include an unpleasant sensation of being mild-headed (though it's nothing like feeling excessive) dry mouth and a drop in blood pressure. There are many individuals out there who have their blood pressure decreased should not be considered as a negative result.

There are a few side negative effects that may occur. If you are pregnant, or are currently nursing the baby may not wish to take a shot of CBD oil. There's no evidence that this could be dangerous to the expecting baby, or the mother. However, there is no reliable evidence for the degree of safe it could be also. The fact that is acknowledged is that it's commonplace for a variety of herbal remedies to harm mothers who are nursing or expecting.

One area in which CBD oil isn't suggested, as its side negative effects could make matters more difficult for people suffering from Parkinson's. A lot of people with Parkinson's disease say that CBD oil helps them get more sleep and manage fewer spasms and increased control over their movements more effectively. On the other side that spectrum just the opposite is true as well. Some people who utilized CBD oil as a result of Parkinson's disease have stated that it's made the tremors they experience at night and their muscle movement while they sleep even more difficult. As more evidence is required on the results of CBD oil for Parkinson's disease, it might be beneficial to seek alternatives to fight the disease other than CBD oil.

Dosage quantity

CBD oil isn't difficult to track, but some individuals use it routinely and do not pay attention to the amount they consume. It is a common practice for those who smoke it. Mixing it with food and water, adhere to the instructions included in the recipe or check the water bottle for the dosage recommended. Take care to follow the directions on any tablet which can be placed in the mouth or swallowed. If you are using CBD oil for specific medical reasons 300 milligrams daily is the dose recommended. The amount of CBD oil could be used for up to six months without dealing with backlash. To get higher doses in CBD oil, around 1,200 to 1,500 milligrams per day, you should only make use of CBD oil for a maximum of CBD oil for a period of 4 weeks prior to having a rest from it. For issues that are more fragile you should consult your physician for the best quantity of CBD oil you must be taking, as well as the length of time you need using the product.

Given that you've done very well in reading this far and because we're assuming that you're eager to dive directly into the process of using CBD rather than reading the entire text right from the beginning A comprehensive and easy-to-use guide has been prepared to provide you with short guideline to provide an answer to a few most frequently asked CBD oil-related queries.

Who were the trailblazers who made the path to CBD oil to be used for medical purposes?

Roger Adams

Dr. Walter S. Loewe

Dr. Ralph Mechoulam

There is a chance that you're wondering whether knowing who these people are important when you get in the habit of taking CBD oil. The truth is it's not necessary to know their identities to take pleasure in

CBD or to reap many advantages. Knowing and comprehend any subject however small it may appear at first glance, it can be a significant way to bind you with any practice or product that you are interested in. Understanding who they are is as well as revealing the inverse side of your life you might not have noticed. The stifling of your mind by ponderous musings won't be an option, however it's a good idea to remember that when you attempt to go on a trip and escape from the irony of medical practice today It is important to remember that those have discovered and harvested the CBD oil that you plan to utilize were created by experts.

Strange as it is it is, in reality, science is the reflection of the natural world and there's an exchange of information between humans and nature. Be aware that doctors and scientists do not have to be opponents. Technology is not a part of nature, personality as well as no moral code. It is not limited to cars, phones and laptops however, all medicines both natural and other also. It's the way technology is utilized by both males and females that will determine what is truly valuable about something. This is true for CBD oil. It would be a good idea to keep in mind the fact that CBD oil also is a form of technology. It may be derived out of nature but the process of it as well as the different methods used to use it bear the hallmarks of the modern age written over them.

What are the many ways to ensure that CBD oil is in the human body?

CBD oil is a great ingredient to mix in with water or incorporated into specific food items. When you cook your food using olive oil, you can add some CBD oil to your dish before enjoying your dinner.

CBD is a sublingual drug that can be consumed this means CBD is able to be administered beneath the tongue.

CBD oil may be used in tablets which resemble pills. This is a simple procedure for people who are just beginning to use CBD or those looking to change their CBD usage to be similar to the modern-day medicines.

CBD oil is applied as a spray can be sprayed on the mouth.

Inhalation. This is the most frequently utilized method for inhaling CBD oil. CBD oil. It is more sophisticated and might not be the best choice for people who are just beginning their journey. However, for others, it's not only the most popular method to get CBD oil, but also an extremely popular pastime that could be a way to enter an entirely new group of friends. There is a wide range of flavors and gadgets that are used to vape and you'll need to take your time and conduct some additional study before diving into the water of inhaling CBD oil.

The topical application can also be utilized. Everyone ought to try at least one time before making a an ultimate verdict on it. If CBD oil is utilized in the form of a lotion or cream it's effects are immediately. There are numerous smells and scents associated with the use of CBD oil in topical application. Utilizing CBD oil this way could also open the door to the realm of cosmetics and skincare, should you be interested in exploring that area, or already believed you were an integral part of the process.

Be aware that you may at any time add CBD oil to your bath. If you choose to add a tiny amount or even a full bath bomb with CBD oil, however you choose to do it you'll be able to enjoy to enjoy a soothing bath.

What are the various types of oil that originate from the Cannabis indica plant?

CBD oil

Oil extracted from hemp seeds

Marijuana oil

THC oil

Cannabis oil

What are the ailments that CBD oil could be utilized to cure?

Acne

Epilepsy

Insomnia

Anxiety

Stress

Depression

PTSD

Chron's illness

Ulcerative colitis

Glaucoma

Chapter 7: What Is Cannabidiol (Cbd)?

CBD is the acronym for cannabidiol and is the second-most abundant cannabinoid in the hemp plant and has many potential therapeutic benefits, including anti-inflammatory, analgesic, anti-anxiety and seizure-suppressant properties just to name a few. It can be sourced from both marijuana plants and hemp plants, which are legal in most countries as they contain minor amounts of THC.

CBDis one of the most well-known chemical compounds found inside the cannabis plant aside from THC. Unlike THC however, CBD does not produce the psychoactive effect that has become commonly associated with marijuana nor many of the other symptoms. In other words, they are both cannabinoids, but one is distinctly separate from THC meaning that they are different substances.CBD is also extremely famous for its ability to reduce the side effects of THC.

Because of its non-psychoactive effects and great potential healing properties, cannabidiol holds an exceptionally high medicinal value that will be paramount in how we treat medical conditions moving forward. It has unique traits that make it stand out as an excellent treatment for a variety of conditions, symptoms, and diseases.

CBD is found in both hemp and cannabis

Hemp is a variety of the Cannabis Sativa plant that is grown for the industrial use of its fiber.Its history dates back over 10,000 years and is used to provide the raw material for textiles, biodegradable plastics, rope, nutraceuticals, construction materials, biofuel, food and more. Hemp is a tall, non-psychoactive plant, containing low levels of THC.

Note: For the purposes of this book, "marijuana" and "cannabis" will be used interchangeably even though we know that hemp is also a cannabis plant.

At the time the Controlled Substances Act of 1970 went into effect, it was illegal to grow industrial hemp in the United States. However, hemp products that werelegally sold in the US had to meet three criteria:

The hemp could not originate in the U.S.

It must've been lawfully imported

The material must've been derived from the "mature stalks and seeds" or "oil and cake made from seeds" of industrial hemp plants.

CBD products sold in states where medical/recreational marijuana is legal can extract CBD from either industrial hemp or a CBD-rich strain of cannabis.However, there are notable differences between CBD derived from cannabis versus hemp.

The synergy of the different compounds in cannabis work together to produce therapeutic effects on the body that are not achieved by the compounds individually. Essentially, the compounds work better together in what is known as the 'entourage effect.' Because of this, CBD derived from cannabis can be more effective when administered with higher levels of THC and terpenes. The mixture of the compounds accentuates the desired effects of cannabinoids on the body. For example, clinical research has shown that a 1:1 ratio of CBD to THC is effective for neuropathic pain.

As a whole, industrial hemp still contains less CBD than CBD-rich cannabis strains and lacks the robust terpene and cannabinoid profile that cannabis provides. Large amounts of industrial hemp are required to extract a small amount of CBD oil, raising questions about contaminants. Hemp is a bioaccumulator, meaning it draws toxins from the soil that could potentially end up in the extracted oil. This is one reason you want to make sure that the brand of CBD you decide to purchase has been properly tested.

CBD is best extracted from the flower and leaves, and only to a minor extent, the stalk of the hemp plant.

CBD oil and products that are obtained from the Cannabis sativa plant or more specifically, industrial hemp,contain high amounts of CBD and only trace amounts THC.

This means that hemp extract containing hemp CBD is ideal for those wishing to harness its powerful effects. Other hemp products include hemp oil, which is a healthy addition to a balanced diet and a nurturing addition to skincare and hair products.

How CBD works?

Despite the fact that there are all kinds of studies and intense research is being performed about the ways that CBD works in the body, this is not entirely clear yet. What scientists do know for a fact is that CBD, just like THC, causes a broad range of effects in our bodies by interacting with the endocannabinoid system which includes two types of cannabinoid receptors: CB1 and CB2.

CB1 receptors can be found in many areas of the brain, and they play an essential role in functions such as mood, memory, sleep, pain sensation, and appetite.

CB2 receptors are usually found in the immune system are they are responsible for cannabis' anti-inflammatory effects.

Endocannabinoids (cannabinoids produced by the body)typically activate both CB1 and CB2 receptors, and the main endocannabinoids that are found in our body are anandamide and arachidonoyl glycerol.The Endocannabinoid System is a vital system in the human body, which has receptors spread out across the entire organism, with higher concentrations in the brain and immune system. This system has evolved to specifically manage the effects of cannabinoids in the body, such as THC and CBD.

When CBD enters the body, the ECS receptors pick up on these compounds and immediately react and start regulating and managing them to where they are most needed and can do the most good. By sending these compounds in the areas of the body which need them the most, the ECS is actively working to induce a state of balance in the organism, and boost overall health.

With receptors all over the human body, the Endocannabinoid System controls vital functions such as pain, inflammation, sleep, mood, memory, appetite, and more. When you stimulate the Endocannabinoid System with CBD supplements, it will, in turn, regulate and improve vital functions in your body, with little to no health risks or side effects.

THC mimics the effects of the body's endocannabinoids by also activating both CB1 and CB2 receptors. But, unlike THC, CBD doesn't seem to act directly on cannabinoid receptors. Instead, it works indirectly on them, and it boosts the levels of endocannabinoids in the body. CBD can stimulate the release of endocannabinoids, and it also interferes with their natural breakdown.

Main effects of CBD

Anti-depressant: It combats anxiety and depression.

Anti-convulsant: It suppresses seizure activity.

Anti-oxidant: It fights neuro-degenerative disorders.

Anti-psychotic: It combats psychosis.

Neuro-protective: It protects the neurons in the brain.

Anti-emetic: It reduces nausea and vomiting.

Anti-inflammatory: It combats inflammation and also the pain.

Anti-tumoral: It combats tumor and cancer cells.

How THC works?

When THC penetrates the brain, it stimulates the cells to release the substance called dopamine, and it also activates the cannabinoid receptors which affect the brain in various ways. The initial state will be a relaxed one combined with a mellow feeling. The eyes may dilate, and other senses will be enhanced. More reported effects include a mix of emotions such as happiness and elation, unease and anxiety, relaxation and pain relief.

When cannabis is smoked, the THC (tetrahydrocannabinol) enters the bloodstream and makes its way to the brain where it interferes with receptors. The largest numer of these receptors reside in the par of the brain that controlspleasure, memory, concentration, sensory experiences, time perception, learning and coordination.

THC will also change the way we think. It can also cause hallucinations and delusions. The immediate effects usually start within 10 to 30 minutes after THC consumption.

Main effects of THC

Analgesic: It relieves pain and inflammation.

Relaxation: It creates a state of relaxation and well-being.

Drowsiness: It induces sleep.

Euphoria: It causes the state of "high."

Appetite stimulant: It creates the urge to eat.

The psychoactive/psychological effects of THC include the following: time distortion, intensified sensory experiences, increased socialization.

CBD lacks all these harmful cognitive effects featured by THC, and in fact, it can even counteract the psychoactive effects of THCwhen administered from the extract and in plant form.

Medicinal properties of CBD

As you can see, CBD has "multiple targets of action," meaning that it works at many different places, giving it numerous medicinal properties, which include:

Potent anti-inflammatory

Antioxidant

Neuroprotectant

Anticonvulsant

Analgesic (pain reliever)

Anxiolytic (anti-anxiety)

Antidepressant

Antipsychotic

Antispasmodic

Anti-cancer agent

CBD modulates the intoxicating effects of THC and reduces the adverse effects that some people experience with THC, namely rapid heartbeat, anxiety, and short-term memory loss. At the same time, when CBD is taken with THC to treat pain, the combination reduces pain more significantly than THC alone. In low doses, CBD is described as alerting. In high doses it can be sedating. Amazingly, CBD has very little side effects even at high doses.

Common health benefits of CBD

Scientific research shows the many health benefits ofCBD. Even despiteCBD being a component of marijuana, it does not produce the psychoactive effects that have made marijuana attractive for recreational use. CBD benefits are real because CBD produces strong medicinal and therapeutic effects for even the most common conditions.

Digestive Aid

A healthy appetite is vital to a healthy body, especially when the body is healing. Some illnesses decrease the appetite to the point of preventing the body from healing itself. CBD stimulates appetite, according to the National Cancer Institute. In the human body, CBDs bind to cannabinoid receptors in the body. Scientists believe these receptors play an important role in regulating feeding behavior.

CBD also eases nausea and vomiting. This is especially helpful for individuals enduring chemotherapy and other treatments for serious diseases.

Analgesic

CBDs affect the CB1 receptors in the body to relieve pain. CBD also has an anti-inflammatory effect that reduces swelling that would be associated with the CB2 receptor.

Anxiety Relief

CBD may alleviate severe social anxiety. Generalized Social Anxiety Disorder (SAD), is one of the most common forms of anxiety disorders that impair quality of life. Some consumers complain of increased social anxiety after marijuana use, but this may be due to low levels of CBD proportionate to the higher levels of THC.

Scientists wanted to study the effects of CBD on people with SAD. The scientists selected 24 people with this condition who had never received treatment for SAD, then divided participants into two groups. One group received 600 mg of CBD while the control group received a placebo. The scientists then asked study participants to take part in a simulated public speaking test while researchers measured blood pressure, heart rate and other measurements of physiological and psychological stress.

The CBD group showed significantly reduced anxiety, cognitive impairment and discomfort in their speech performance. In comparison, those in the placebo group presented higher anxiety, cognitive impairment and discomfort.

According to the National Institute of Mental Health, approximately 15 million adults in the United States have social phobia and about 6.8 million have a generalized anxiety disorder. Traditional treatment usually involves counseling and medications. Treatment with CBD may be better than anti-depressants because it acts quickly and does not cause side effects or withdrawal symptoms.

Cancer Spread

The National Cancer Institute details several studies into the anti-tumor effects of CBD. One study in mice and rats suggest CBDs "may have a protective effect against the development of certain types of tumors." CBDs may do this by inducing tumor cell death, inhibiting cancer cell growth, and by controlling and inhibiting the spread of cancer cells.

One study by California Pacific Medical Center suggests CBD "turns off" the gene involved in the spread of breast cancer. These scientists found CBD inhibits ID-1, an action that prevents cancer cells from traveling long distances to distant tissues.

How does CBDinteract with the body?

All of the 60 plus cannabinoids unique to the plant genuscannabis, interact with our bodies through the endocannabinoid system.

If you recall, the endocannabinoid system runs throughout your body. It's loaded with receptors that bind to the cannabinoids you introduce to your bloodstream when you consume cannabis. It's the chemical interactions of those bonds that create a wide and largely unknown series of responses in your body.

And even though CBD has no psychoactivefor humans, meaning, it doesn't make you intoxicated (i.e. high), it is highly reactive with the endocannabinoid system.

To put things as simply as possible, CBD makes things happen. When it interactswith the endocannabinoid system's receptors, it stimulates all kinds of changes in the body.

Where does cbd come from?

Cannabis plants come in a variety of strains. Each strain produces a particular balance of cannabinoids. Cannabinoids can account for as much as 25% or more of the content of the flowers. The amount of cannabinoids a plant can produce is limited, so as one cannabinoid is bred into a strain, the others are bred out. So, there are strains that are high in THC and low in CBD, and others that are high in CBD and low in THC, and some plants have more of a balance of the two.

Some strains of hemp are bred to be high in CBD and extremely low in THC. The essential oil extracts of cannabis flowers contain cannabinoids in the same ratio as the plant from which it is extracted, therefore, hemp extracts contain negligible amounts of THC.

Hemp is also far cheaper to grow and process than marijuana, so quite often, the CBD in CBD-infused products is extracted from hemp rather than marijuana and refined into CBD-rich essential oils and pure CBD. In order for a patient to be sure that their medicine is 100% THC-free, only hemp-derived products should be used. Note: Hemp plants do contain trace amounts of THC (<0.3%).

Chapter 8: How Is Cbdmade?

In order to extract CBD from the hemp plant, the flowers and leaves are ground up and soaked in a solvent of some kind (ethanol, supercritical CO_2, etc.) which separates the essential oils from the plant matter. The resulting product is correctly referred to as hemp extract. This extract will contain cannabinoids and other oily compounds found in the plant such as terpenes in the same ratio as the plant.

The next step in producing CBD is to concentrate the extract using a distillation process. This removes some of the unwanted contents and produces CBD concentrate. The resulting ratio of CBD and other compounds depends on the process and how many steps of distillation it has gone through.

CBD concentrate can also be further refined to produce CBD isolate, which can be as high as 99% pure CBD. CBD isolate takes on a salt-like crystal form at room temperature.

CBD concentrates and CBD isolates can be consumed by themselves, or they can be added to vegetable oils such as hemp seed oil, coconut oil, olive oil, and so on, as well as non-plant-based oils such as emu oil. These preparations can be used both internally and topically.

IS CBD LEGAL?

Is CBD legal? This is the most common, and most misunderstood, question surrounding this subject. There used to be a time that CBD and THC were both classified by the Drug Enforcement Agency (DEA) as Schedule 1 drug at the federal level. That means that the US federal government classified these two substances under the same schedule that includes Heroin, LSD, and Ecstacy, just to name a few of the more common ones.

The history of cannabis goes back thousands of years and is an excellent subject for future writings, but we're going to concentrate on the part of history when cannabis first started being regulated in the United States.

Here's a timeline to help you better understand some of the contemporary history of cannabis:

Up until 1906 – Cannabis, including hemp, was a primary crop grown by thousands of farmers including some of our forefathers like George Washington, Thomas Jefferson, and John Adams.

1906 – Restrictions started increasing.

1920s – Prohibitions began.

Mid – 1930s - Cannabis was being regulated as a drug in every state, not to mention the 35 states that adopted the Uniform State Narcotic Drug Act which was primarily to produce revenue for the federal government.

1937 – First regulation of cannabis came about with the Marihuana Tax Act of 1937.

1970 – The Controlled Substances Act of 1970 was officially passed and formally outlawed the use of cannabis for any use, including medical.

On December 20, 2018, President Donald Trump signed into law the Agriculture Improvement Act of 2018 (more commonly known as the 2018 Farm Bill). The 2018 Farm Bill, which went into effect on January 1, 2019, contains a broad range of provisions but among them are the legalization of the cultivation and sale of hemp. As a result of the 2018 Farm Bill, hemp is no longer classified as a Schedule 1 substance. Keep in mind that the Farm Bill is a federal statute and only legalizes hemp (and as a result, CBD made from hemp) at thefederal level. So, while CBD is legal under Federal Law, it is always prudent to check your local laws.

The best way for manufacturers to avoid legal issues is to extract the CBD from hemp rather than cannabis. Some stores use industrial hemp grown by US farmers and processed in pharmaceutical grade facilities.

In the United States, any variety of cannabis with a THC concentration of not more than 0.3% is considered to be 'industrial hemp.' So as long as the CBD that you're using comes from hemp and contains less than 0.3% THC, you shouldn't have any concerns.

States where CBD is legal for recreational use

As of the writing of this book there are 10states where the cannabis plant, including both marijuana and hemp are completely legal for recreational and medicinal use. These states, including Washington DC, are:

Alaska

California

Colorado

Maine

Massachusetts

Michigan

Nevada

Oregon

Vermont

Washington

So if you find yourself in one of these awesome states, you are free to legally use CBD in any form without regard to THC levels and without a prescription.

States where CBD is legal for medicinal use

In addition to the ten states that have legalized recreational marijuana, there are 23 other states that it is legal, but only at the medicinal level. These states include:

Arizona

Arkansas

Connecticut

Deleware

Florida

Hawaii

Illinois

Louisiana

Maryland

Minnesota

Missouri

Montana

New Hampshire

New Jersey

New Mexico

New York

North Dakota

Ohio

Oklahoma

Pennsylvania

Rhode Island

Utah

West Virginia

We just listed a total of 33 states that some form of marijuana is legal and as a result, CBD as well. There are a total of 14 states that have some form of legal CBD at the medicinal level that doesn't fall into a list as nicely as the states listed above. They are:

Alabama – The only way to get CBD legally in Alabama is to be a part of a state sponsored clinical trial or have a debilitating medical condition.

Georgia – A patient can have CBD prescribed in Georgia providing the patient has at least one of over a dozen medical conditions. These medical conditions include cancer, Parkinson's disease, multiple sclerosis, and seizure disorders. The patient can't have more than 20 ounces of oil. The oil cannot be more than 5% THC and the CBD content must be greater than or equal to the THC content. In otherwords, for CBD oil to be legal in Georgia, it must contain at least as much CBD as it does THC.

Indiana–Early in 2018, Indiana moved away from only allowing citizens that was on its patient registry to buy and use CBD oil. On March 21, 2018, the Governor of Indiana signed into law Senate Enrolled Act 52, which legalized the manufacturing, retail sell, and use of CBD oil provided it did not exceed 0.3% THC content in it.

Iowa – The Department of Public Health will allow patients to use limited amounts of CBD oil as long as they are suffering from a predetermined list of medical conditions such as cancer, HIV/AIDS, seizures, and ALS.

Kansas – An adult in Kansas can legally purchase, possess, and use CBD products as long as it doesn't contain any THC whatsoever.

Kentucky–Even though there is growing support for the legalization of marijuana and CBD at least at the medical level, Kentucky can't seem to break away from the legislation they passed in 2014 which revised the definition of marijuana to create legal protection for patients who use CBD.

Mississippi – The current CBD laws in Mississippi was adopted in 2014. The law makes it legal for patients with severe epilepsy to use CBD. The extract must have more than 15% CBD and no more than 0.5% THC. Patients that are prescribed CBD in Mississippi must consume it under the supervision of a licensed physician.

NorthCarolina – North Carolina does have a medical cannabis program set to end in 2021 if studies fail to show and prove the benefits of CBD. As it stands now, patients with intractable epilepsy have access to low THC hemp extract.

SouthCarolina – CBD is legal only to those patients suffering from severe epilepsy. The extract must be at least 15% CBD and no more than 0.9% THC.

Tennessee – Again, only patients diagnosed with intractable epilepsy may be prescribed a CBD extract. It must not contain more than 0.9% THC. Only CBD extracted fromfrom the hemp plant is legal in Tennessee.

Texas –The Compassionate Use Act only allows patients diagnosed with epileptic seizures by a doctor who specializes in epilepsy to prescribe CBD. The CBD extract prescribed must not have more than 0.5% THC.The caveat is, the patient must try two current FDA approved epilepsy drugs before they can be prescribed CBD.

Virginia–CBD oil is legal for any patient who has any condition that has been diagnosed by a licensed doctor or practitioner.

Wisconsin – In 2014 CBD was only legal to treat seizure disorders. In 2017, the Wisconsin Senate expanded the legal parameters to include the treatment of any medical condition a doctor has recommended it for.

Wyoming – CBD is only legal for patients with epilepsy. Again, the patient must not have responded favorably to other treatments. Even then, a neurologist must plead a case with the Wyoming Department of Health on how CBD would in fact help the patient. The extract will be high concentrations of CBD with trace amounts of THC.

The push to legalize cannabis started in 1996 when California voted to legalize it for medicinal purposes. To date, a total of 47 states have adopted legal cannabis laws of some sort, ranging from purchasing CBD with zero THC to full legalization of recreational marijuana and everything in between. Three states still haven't adopted any laws allowing adults to purchase cannabis in any way, shape, or form. They are:

Idaho

South Dakota

Nebraska

State and federal laws are constantly changing around cannabis. If you live in a state where the cannabis laws are a little gray, I highly recommend you familiarize yourself with the laws of your state.

DOES CBD GET YOU HIGH?

There are dozens of chemicals in the cannabis flower that have very different effects; some of them have no real effect, but others can change your perception on the way medical marijuana is used.

CBD and THC are the most popular known cannabinoids which form a group of chemical compounds that are naturally produced only by cannabis plants. Both CBD and THC exist in the crystalline resinous trichomes that cover the mature cannabis flower, and both of them are the cannabinoids that we find most abundantly in marijuana. But each strain produces different amounts of the compounds. They share the same chemical formula with the only difference is that their atoms are arranged in a variety of ways, but they have widely different effects on our body because they interact with our endocannabinoid system differently.

CBD does not get you high. In fact, when taken with THC, CBD actually reduces just how high you can get. Here's the science behind why CBD won't get you high and how it takes the edge off the high produced by THC.

Think of THC and CBD as batteries. THC is a AA, and CBD is a AAA. The CB1 receptor in your brain only turns on when the right size battery is inserted, in this case, the AA

(THC). The AA fits nicely into the receptor, turns it on, and produces the psychoactive high that we have all heard of and/or experienced.

But the AAA (CBD) also fits into the receptor. It's not an exact match like the AA, so the AAA doesn't activate the receptor. That's why CBD doesn't get you high: it's not built to activate the receptors that cause your world to go psychedelic.

So now you've got an AAA battery occupying a space made for an AA battery. If an AA battery comes along, it's going to "bounce off" that receptor because the AAA battery is already there. That's how CBD can take the edge off the high caused by THC: the CBD molecule reduces the chances that THC will activate the CB1 receptors. In essence, it's a clash between cannabinoids.

ARE THERE ANY RISKS OR SIDE EFFECTS?

Although, side effects are very rare to those consuming CBD,it's important to note that the impact of the few that do exist could be unwelcome. Take drowsiness for example. If taken in tandem with a medication that also causes drowsiness, patients who must be alert for work could be put at risk.

So far, CBD has not been shown to have any severe or fatal impact on patients in clinical trials. Here are a few of the minor CBD side effects that could be unwelcome for potential consumers of the medication.

Impacts on drug metabolism

The body produces a series of enzymes that help patients to consume and benefit from CBD. Use of CBD combined with other drugs can keep medications from being properly processed by the body.

In test trials, CBD has been shown to neutralize P450 enzyme activity in some patients. This is one of the main enzymes in the liver that helps to metabolize medications. This should remind patients to consult a physician or a pharmacist before adding any medications to their routine. It should be noted that grapefruits can also have this impact on the liver's metabolizing capabilities. So no need to panic if you've taken CBD in tandem with any medication. But it's important to check and see if your medication is still working. Complications like these can easily be worked out by rescheduling your medication at different times of the day. You can live with a reduced P450 enzyme for a short time as your body can reset the balance a few hours later.

Dry mouth

If you have issues with dehydration, CBD could exacerbate your problems. Some patients have reported CBD side effects that include an 'unpleasant dry sensation throughout the day.' As noted above, CBD has an effect on secretions of glands and this will include saliva. Cannabinoid receptors are present in the glands that produce saliva, which can lead to dry mouth. It's not too severe of an impact but can cause some amount of discomfort. Staying hydrated or drinking sports drinks with electrolytes can counteract this balance.

It could have the positive impact of getting some patients to drink more water than they normally would on a given day.

Increased tremors

For people who suffer from Parkinson's disease, CBD should not be taken in high doses. High doses in some early research has been shown to increase tremors for Parkinson's patients. Inflammation and pain related to Parkinson's can be treated with CBD. Many patients report positive impacts on the other effects of Parkinson's.

When taken in lower doses, CBD has been tested to having positive impacts on alleviating Parkinson's related pain. If you're taking CBD related to Parkinson's, your CBD side effects could be a dosage issue. Try lowering the dosage before discarding the treatment altogether. Always consult your doctor before beginning any treatment or changing your dosage.

Low blood pressure

As CBD slows down some of the body's processes during moments of inflammation or illness, it can also work to slow the process too much. CBD could cause a drop in blood pressure for some patients. It usually happens right after you administer the medication.

Low blood pressure can be an issue if you're recovering from surgery or any kind of accident. It also affects how quickly other medications will move through your system.

If you experience any of the lightheadedness often associated with low blood pressure, talk to a physician. It could be an effect of your CBD treatment or a drug interaction you may not have predicted.

As we've said before, the side effects associated with CBD are virtually non esistent to the vast majority of consumers using it. However, it's always a good idea to consult a medical professional before embarking on your first CBD journey.

Chapter 9: What Are Terpenes?

Terpenes are basically the unsaturated hydrocarbons found in the essential oils of plants. They are found in different plants and even some insects. When you walk through a forest and smell the pine scent in the air, you are essentially smelling the terpene Pinene, which is responsible for giving you that uplifting feeling. Another example is the smell of lemon when you're polishing your furniture. The terpene Limonene can be thanked for that smell and the good mood that comes with it. Although there are literally hundreds of terpenes in nature, there are only about ten that really affect the world of cannabis. They are:

Pinene

Limonene

Myrcene

Linalool

Delta-3-Carene

Eucalyptol

Caryophyllene

Humulene

Ocimene

Terpineol

The following is an in depth look at the ten most commonly found terpenes in the cannabis plant. You will find that all these terpenes have an aroma associated with it, as well as certain health benefits, different vaporizing temperatures, various medicinal values, and different places to find each of them in nature.

A closer look at common terpenes in cannabis

Pinene

Smells like pine

Vaporizes at 311 degrees F.

Used to treat asthma, pain, ulcers, anxiety, and cancer.

Help with alertness, memory retention, and counteracts some THC effects.

Can be found in pine needles, basil, parsley, dill, and rosemary.

Limonene

Has a citrus smell to it.

Vaporizes at 348 degrees F.

Used to treat anxiety, depression, inflammation, pain, and cancer.

Helps with reducing stress and has a tendency to elevate moods.

Can be found in fruit rinds, rosemary, juniper, and peppermint.

Myrcene

The terpene most prevalent in the cannabis plant.

Concentration dictates whether a strain will have a sedative effect or an energetic effect.

Cardamom, herbal, cloves, musky, and earthy are the aromas for Myrcene. Although a pleasant smell, not one that is used directly too often.

Vaporizes at 332 degrees F.

Used to treat insomnia, pain, inflammation, as well as a great antioxidant.

Helps with relaxation and at levels of >0.5%, can have a sedating "couchlock" effect.

Can be found in mango, lemongrass, thyme, and hops.

Linalool

Has a floral smell

Vaporizes at 388 degrees F.

Used to treat anxiety, depression, insomnia, pain, inflammation, and neurodegeneration.

Helps with sedation and mood enhancement.

Found in lavender.

Delta-3-Carene

Has a sweet, pungent, woody, pine, and cedar combination smell.

Vaporizes at 338 degrees F.

Used to treat depression, and is a good anti-inflammatory and antihistamine. Also used to dry out excess body fluids like sweat, tears, mucus, as well as menstrual flow.

Helps with insomnia and improves memory.

Can be found in pine, cedar, and rosemary.

Eucalyptol

Has a camphor smell to it.

Vaporizes at 349 degrees F.

Used for Alzheimer's, asthma, bacteria, cancer, anti-oxidant, and anti-inflammatory.

Helps with mental clarity and headaches.

Can be found in eucalyptus, camphor laurel, bay leaves, tea tree, mugwort, sweet basil, wormwood, rosemary, and common sage.

Caryophyllene

Smells like cloves and pepper as well as spicy and woody.

Vaporizes at 266 degrees F.

Used for pain, anxiety, depression, and ulcers.

Helps with stress relief.

Found in black pepper, cloves, and cinnamon.

Humulene

Has a woody, earthy aroma with the smell of hops

Vaporizes at 222 degrees F.

Used primarily as an anti-inflammatory.

Found in coriander, basil, cloves, and hops.

Ocimene

Smells sweet, herbal, and woody.

Vaporizes at 122 degrees F.

Used for antiviral, antifungal, antibacterial, antiseptic, and a decongestant.

Found in basil, mangoes, orchids, pepper, parsley, mint, and kumquats.

Terpineol

Aroma is piney, floral, and herbal.

Vaporizes at 366 degrees F.

Used for cancer, fungus, bacteria, sedative, and an antioxidant.

Has a sedating effect.

Found in nutmeg, apples, conifers, tea tree, lilacs, and cumin.

Keep in mind that since CBD isolates are stripped down to just the CBD, they lack most, if not all, of the terpenes that is naturally found in the plant. I'm not saying that the CBD isolates are not a good option, especially if THC is a factor. What I am saying is that you can't get the entourage effect of the CBD through an isolate.

FULL SPECTRUM VS ISOLATE

Due to its non-psychoactive healing properties, CBD has become a very popular option for patients seeking a natural alternative to treat conditions such as chronic pain, anxiety, epilepsy, and more. As patients start to understand how CBD can be used to alleviate their symptoms, they are often faced with a choice between using products made from CBD isolate or full spectrum CBD.

Difference between CBD isolate vs full spectrum CBD

When CBD is referred to as full spectrum or whole plant CBD, it means that the CBD contains all the other cannabinoids found in the cannabis or hemp plant (about 85 total) including CBN (Cannabinol), CBG (Cannabigerol), and THCV (Tetrahydrocannabivarin), to name a few. THC and CBD are the ones we are most familiar with. Full spectrum CBD from hemp contains trace amounts of THC but in very low concentrations (up to 0.3%). Full spectrum CBD from the cannabis plant can contain significantly higher amounts of THC.

CBD isolate, on the other hand, is simply purified CBD that has been extracted from the cannabis or hemp plant and isolated from the other cannabinoids. So essentially, it's CBD in its purest form without any other cannabinoids to accompany it.

CBD isolate vs full spectrum CBD: Which is more effective?

It was previously believed that CBD in its isolated form was more potent and concentrated than full spectrum CBD. However, in 2015, the theory was debunked by a study from the Lautenberg Center for General Tumor Immunology in Jerusalem. In the study, researchers administered full spectrum CBD and CBD isolate to two different groups of mice. When comparing the data of the two groups, the results proved that the group administered with full spectrum CBD were provided with higher levels of relief. Furthermore, the study demonstrated that full spectrum CBD continued to provide relief as the dose increased, while CBD isolate did not provide the same effect when there was an increase in dosage.

While full spectrum CBD has ultimately proven to be more effective than CBD isolate and can be used to effectively treat a wide variety of ailments, it does not discredit the effectiveness of CBD isolate.

There are a wide variety of situations when CBD isolate would be preferred over full spectrum CBD. For example, you may not necessarily need the full capabilities of full spectrum CBD, or if you aren't legally allowed to use THC. It is also important to note that other cannabinoids may cause negative reactions when isolated CBD wouldn't (if the condition you are suffering from is critical, weadvise you speak to a medical consultant before trying out any version of CBD).

Products that advertise "whole plant CBD" are also good because they'll incorporate the entourage effect. The entourage effect refers to how cannabinoids and terpenes react with one another in the body. Research suggests that these compounds work best when combined together like they are naturally found in the marijuana plant, rather than if they are isolated in a lab. Therefore, whole plant CBD products are usually more effective than CBD isolates.

CBD AS AN ANTI-INFLAMMATORY

The anti-inflammatory properties of CBD come well documented. Reducing inflammation is a recognized potential use case for the diverse cannabinoid. Naturally, reducing inflammation helps to combat chronic inflammation. Believed to be the precursor to heart disease, diabetes, and several forms of cancer, chronic inflammationprevention is linked to living a longer, happier life.

In one study, they monitored the reaction between CBD and glycine receptors. The receptors were linked to dorsal horn neurons in the spines of rats. These are a collection of sensory neurons that transmit information,in this case telling our brain we are in pain. Researchers concluded that administration of CBD, significantly suppress chronic inflammatory and neuropathic pain.

A further studyexamined the effectiveness of CBD at mitigating inflammation. The study focussed on biopsies from patients with ulcerative colitis (UC) and intestinal segments of mice with LPS-induced intestinal inflammation. UC is a long-term chronic condition that causes the human colon and rectum to become inflamed. Again, CBD demonstrated its efficiency. Preliminary results showed that CBD counteracts the inflammatory environment induced by LPS in mice and also in human colonic cultures derived from UC patients.

CBD can reduce inflammation too much

Thankfully, that is something scientists at the Research Center of the University Institute of Cardiology and Pulmonology of Quebec also wanted to understand. An appropriate inflammatory response is vital for our immune system to be effective in fighting infections. By analysing data collated by the scientific community, the regulation of lung immunity and inflammation caused by cannabinoids was scrutinized.

Initial interpretation found that through the downregulation of the functions of immune cells, cannabinoids could diminish host defence. Doing so would increase the risk of contracting an infection, and reduce our immune system's effectiveness. They did go on to acknowledge that the relationship between too much and too little support with inflammation is a complicated one. More extensive research would be needed to transfer the data from animal models to humans.

Too much of a good thing can be bad

Conflicting research always makes for concerned reading. However, the inflammatory "balancing act" is no different from several other aspects of healthy living. If you take a look in your medicine cabinet, it is bound to be filled with a broad spectrum of health supplements. Iron, vitamin D, vitamin C; several essential supplements are needed to give our bodies a boost. It is a form of support that may be needed because of limitations in lifestyle or diet. Just like the scenario with CBD, ingesting too many vitamins can lead to adverse effects.

We shouldn't fear the implications of taking too much of something that is good for us. In most cases, the tolerable level is much higher when the effect is beneficial, rather than detrimental. In reality, something that is "good" for us can be "bad," and vice versa. The trouble is, if we segregate products in this way, it becomes impossible to know if a supplement is safe to consume. Instead, we should always come back to the theme of balance. Good versus bad is merely too basic, especially when each of us is uniquely different in our genetic makeup.

Dosage is crucial

We know from research that CBD has fantastic potential as a potent anti-inflammatory. We also know that in some of the data collected, this can lead to diminished effectiveness in our immune system. Presented with those two statements, the next logical step is to factor in dosage. The ideal dose of CBD will depend on numerous variables,more than have been studied thus far. Your physiology, the condition or disease, CBD concentration, external factors; the list of potential parameters is extensive.

While we wait for the experts to identify and narrow down variables, the safest option is to start low. Build CBD intake slowly to establish the impact on your own body. With a little patience, the hope is that comprehensive research will establish and quantify the exact implications of CBD use.

How can CBD be used as an anti-inflammatory drug?

Of all the qualities that CBD offers, it's anti-inflammatory properties are arguably the most well researched of the bunch. Being successfully utilized to treat almost all digestive conditions, as well as many other medical challenges, it is now looked upon as the most efficient anti-inflammatory drug available,even beating out traditional options such as Vitamin C and Omega 3 supplements!

It is important to have a good grasp on how CBD works with our bodies, though, in order to fully understand how it can be such a useful anti-inflammatory.

Like all cannabinoids, CBD interacts with our body upon consumption, but what is interesting about CBDis that it works differently to many of the other researched compounds of the plant, particularly when it comes to interaction with the endocannabinoid system.

If you recall, each and every one of us has an Endocannabinoid system (ECS), which has control over regulating many of our bodily functions and ensuring that everything runs smoothly. The ECS releases natural cannabinoids that are vital for a range of physiological things, from the way we think to the way we feel pain. In fact, it plays a part in almost every aspect of our being.

When CBD is consumed, it interacts with the ECS and encourages it to produce an increased number of natural cannabinoids. By doing this, our body is better able to heal and regulate various functions. Also, not only does CBD help produce self healing cannabinoids, but it also interacts with our CB2 receptors, which oversee our entire immune system.

Are you enjoying this book? Are you learning anything? It would really help us out if you could take a minute to leave an honest review. Thank you!

CBD: The Ultimate Oil For Pain Review

Chapter 10: Cbd For Pain Relief

If you're suffering from recurring aches or pains in your body, you know how frustrating it is. Maybe you're struggling through the constant cycle of waking up each morning stiff as a board, or worse yet, in the middle of the night. Is there any relief in sight? If it feels like you're in a constant state of popping anti-inflammatory pills like Aleve or Advil, you might find some relief with CBD oil.

Over the last few years, as CBD oil has become increasingly popular, it's being used to help with pain relief for people of all ages. The difference here is that CBD oil is non-psychoactive, so you're getting the medicinal benefits of cannabis without any of the physical "high."

A lot of medical studies back up the anecdotal claims for CBD's pain relief properties. CBD has properties that bind to the pain receptors within your body. This allows for the body to experience an alleviation in pain.

What causes pain?

Pain might seem to be a nuisance at times, but it is there to serve a purpose. Imagine touching a hot stove. It burns! This pain causes you to quickly retract your finger from what is causing the pain, thereby protecting you. Cuts and scrapes and inflammation that come about from injuries also serve a purpose, with inflammation helping to protect a damaged area and remove pathogens from a wound, preventing infection. The central nervous system exists to alert us to such problems.

How is pain usually treated?

It was once advised that people suffering from chronic pain should stay in bed and rest, but we now know that this is probably the worst thing you can do. If your pain is muscular, such as might be the case with lower back pain, you must keep yourself moving, as staying still for long periods will only stiffen your muscles further. Staying in bed will also stop you from sleeping well, you will become lonely, the pain will get worse, and your other muscles and bones will weaken. It's just not worth it!

Instead, it is important to keep exercising through your pain. This isn't to say you should hit the gym and pump some iron. You can simply walk more, or take part in some swimming (where your weight will be taken by the water), peddle gently on an exercise bike, or engage in yoga. By all means, take and follow the advice of your doctor or physical therapist before working through your pain. But it is a common conception to exercise even despite chronic pain. Many believe that by strengthening the muscles of the body, you are better prepared to combat your pain.

However, this is generally not enough to rid people of chronic pain. Painkillers are extremely common for chronic pain, including over-the-counter medications like aspirin and ibuprofen. These types of medications aren't exactly good for you, though.

First of all, you will only be masking the pain and not solving any of the underlying problems. This is why painkillers such as these need to be taken every 4-6 hours to prevent the pain from returning. But it can be harmful to take these sorts of pharmaceuticals too much, as they can cause stomach ulcers and other damage to the body.

Stronger prescriptions are available for the most serious pains, and this even extends to opioids. Opiate painkillers are very strong and very effective at relieving pain, but they are also extremely addictive. There are literally thousands of overdoses each year in the US.

It's frightening that such a dangerous drug is so widely available for patients, and yet there are much safer and effective options such as CBD.

What type of pain can CBD help with?

We've seen people improve upon all types of pain issues, both chronic and acute pain types. Some of these pain sources include:

Headaches – regular and migranes

Muscle aches

Back pain

Joint pain

Arthritis-related pain

Inflammation relief

I'd like to make it abundantly clear: CBD oil is NOT a miracle cure. You have to give it a try to see if it'll work for you. Everyone's body chemistry is different.A reputable brand won't make outrageous claims about what it can do. It'll simply provide user testimonials and allow you to make the choice.Another important factor to take into consideration is the type of CBD you're using. Some people find that isolates provide the enough relief while others require a full spectrum CBD to find relief.

Although studieson CBD are being done daily, there is still a lot to learn about this very complex topic. With that said, the future is looking bright!

How does CBD work for pain relief?

Unfortunately, pain is a condition of human existence. Everybody experiences pain at one point or another whether it is from a trip or fall, a more serious accident, or if it is caused by an underlying condition, everybody feels pain.

Nowadays, people are looking for alternative methods to treat their aches and pains, as over the counter medications have a long list of drawbacks. Increasingly, CBD is being used for this very matter.

As we learned earlier, the human body contains a network of cannabinoid receptors and endocannabinoids (ones that we produce naturally). The endocannabinoid systemworks to keep our bodies functioning in a healthy manner by maintaining homeostasis, keeping our body in balance.

One of the functions that the ECS helps to regulate is pain and inflammation. It does this by 'listening' to conditions in the body through the cannabinoid receptors that sit on top of each cell. The receptors communicate this information to the inside of the cell, so that different parts of the body can respond accordingly. Hence, when injury occurs, the surrounding area is inflamed to protect it.

As we mentioned though, things can go wrong. If the inflammation persists, it is usually the job of endocannabinoids to stimulate their corresponding receptors to stop it, but this doesn't always happen.

By taking CBD, it is thought that you can indirectly influence the behavior of the ECS. CBD stimulates the production of more endocannabinoids, allowing you to give your body an added boost in times of need. In other words, taking CBD helps your body to work better, naturally.

A review carried out by Dr. Ethan Russo looked at studies ranging from the late 1980s all the way to 2007. Based on the results of these studies, it was concluded that CBD was effective in relieving overall pain without causing any adverse side effects. It was also noted that insomnia caused by chronic pain was relieved. Furthermore, those suffering from pain due to Multiple Sclerosis (MS) were most likely to benefit from CBD use.

From the studies that have been conducted so far, combined with anecdotal evidence from people already using CBD to relieve their pain, it seems that CBD could really offer some hope to people who have to deal with pain in their everyday lives.

CBD oil has a number of medical benefits

For example, studies show that CBD interacts with both your immune system and your brain receptors. These receptors receive a bunch of chemical signals from stimuli and help the rest of your cells respond to those signals. When your receptors react with CBD, they form anti-inflammatory effects that reduce pain.

CBD also helps treat conditions like anxiety, depression, fibromyalgia, and stress.

This makes CBD an effective treatment option for a multitude of medical conditions. But one of the biggest benefits of CBD is that it can help relieve symptoms of chronic pain.

CBD for Chronic Pain

As I've mentioned before, CBD has the ability to interact with the receptors that are found in your brain and also your immune system. So, for example, if you are suffering from chronic back pain, studies and numerous testimonials have have concluded that CBD can help tremendously.You can continuously take CBD oil for your chronic pain and not build up a tolerance to it. In other words, CBD oil provides a long term option for a long term problem. You don't have to keep increasing your dosage or search around for new medications that might work better.

Relieving of arthritis pain

Although many studies still need to be done to better understand painmanagement surrounding arthritis, a great number of arthritis patients have reported significant relief when takingCBD. As I've said before, CBD interacts with two receptors, which are the CB1 and CB2 receptors. The CB2 receptor plays an important role in the immune system and could help explain why CBD might be helpful in patients with inflammatory autoimmune forms of arthritis. A classic example is rheumatoid arthritis.

A recent study, conducted by researchers at the University of Kentucky, investigated the use of CBD in rats with arthritis. In the study, CBD was administered to rats for four consecutive days in the form of a gel, containing either 0.6, 3.1, 6.2, or 62.3 mg. The researchers noticed a reduction in inflammation and overall pain in the rats' arthritic joints, and no side effects were noted.

Cancer treatment

For those that has undergone chemotherapy, they always suffer from pain. But when you take in CBD, there is a good chance that you can manage the pain that might arise due to that painful process.

Relieving of acute pain

When we refer to acute pain, we are referring to pain that is brought onfrom cuts, infections and other kinds of physical injuries that you might get. Acute pain should come and go fast in a few hours, days, or weeks. But this is achievable if you are treated in the right way. As you've already learned, CBD has significant anti-inflammatory properties to it. Pain in general, including various types of acute pain, are caused by the inflammation of the tissue surrounding the injury. So, as a result, the anti-inflammatory properties of CBD can help acute pain.

Fibromyalgia pain

Fibromyalgia is a musculoskeletal disorder that causes pain and as a result, a lack of sleep, headaches, fatigue, depression, muscle pain, memory issues and mood concerns. Pain is a subjective feeling and sometimes it's hard to evaluate and measure it. But research has shown CBD to reduce pain and stiffness, enhance sleep, greater sensation of well-being, and also improvement of relaxation. CBD will give you more options for results with no side effects.

Diabetes pain

If you are suffering from type 1 or even type 2 diabetes, CBD has been shown to reduce inflammation as well as chronic inflammation. It also possesses properties that will improve resistance to insulin. Studies, as well as many testimonials of diabetics, have been shown to lower blood sugar levels, enhance the metabolism of the body and also manage pain from diabetes.

The benefits of using CBD oil for pain relief

CBD has properties that has the ability to work with all types of pain.

Capable of improving swelling, redness, reducing inflammation, and soreness.

It can help you to avoid high doses of Ibuprofen, Oxytocin and also Percocet.

You will not experience any liver or even kidney problems.

If the CBD is in isolate form, the THC level will be so low that it probably will not even show on a drug test.

There are virtually no side effects.

It is not addictive.

It is a natural product.

How to useCBD for pain relief?

There are several ways that you can use to take this product. Some of the ways include:

You can ingest or swallow it.

You can also take it under the tongue, a method known as sublingual.

Consuming it with food or drinks.

CBD is also available in creams which allow you to rub it on your skin.

A brighter future for pain

CBD is a legal compound that can be extracted from the cannabis plant, meaning that oil produced from it is legal to possess and use. More and more people are turning to CBD as a means of relieving symptoms of many conditions, with chronic pain being one of them.

A number of things can cause chronic pain, but no matter what the cause, it is possible that CBD could help. If you are tired of over the counter medications and the risks associated with them, CBD could be a natural way to sootheryour pain and tackle the underlying issue if that is inflammation.

Chapter 11: Cbd For Anxiety

Anxiety affects about 20% of Americans and comes in all shapes and sizes. There are clinical anxiety disorders like social anxiety, PSTD, and OCD, as well as everyday anxieties like trouble sleeping, tight deadlines, and fear of flying.

Many Americans with anxiety disorders are prescribed benzodiazepines like Xanax, Klonopin, and Valium, but these drugs are very addictive and make people feel lethargic and fuzzy.

Anti-anxiety medications have many side effects: cognitive deficits, unusual sleep behaviors, allergic reactions, impairment of driving, decreasing blood pressure, depression, loss of coordination, and increased risk of falling in the elderly. Unlike benzos, CBD has very few possible side effects, and of the few they do have, none are even close to the seriousness of the prescribed medications. Just think, a natural plant with very little possible side effects that produces a substance that helps sufferers with all the classic symptoms of anxiety, like racing thoughts, trouble sleeping, and difficulty being around people.

The other problem with benzodiazepines, they are dangerously addictive. In fact, benzo withdrawal is one of the only withdrawals that could potentially kill. The only other withdrawal as severe is alcohol. Even opioids are less "technically" addictive.

That's why so many people are choosing to quit the "hard stuff" and opt for something more natural, like CBD. In fact, according to a recent State of Cannabis Report by Eaze, 40% of cannabis consumers in California have completely replaced anxiety drugs with cannabis. What's more, of the 48% of respondents that said they use or have used anxiety medication, 95% of them said cannabis has helped them reduce their use of prescription anxiety pills. Those are very significant numbers.

However, because of benzos' highly addictive nature, replacing them with CBD should be done slowly and always, under a medical professional's supervision.

How CBD works for treating anxiety?

Again, CBD interacts with the body's own, natural endocannabinoid system (ECS). You'll notice that we often reference the ECS. The ECS is the core of everything that CBD is to the human body. The ECS is present in nearly "every cell in the body" and helps to regulate many of our bodies' functions, including:

mood

appetite

sleep

memory

pain perception.

In fact, stress recovery is one of the endocannabinoid system's main purposes.

But what's more, researchers described how CBD also interacts with a neurotransmitter called GABA (gamma-aminobutyric acid). GABA transmits messages from one brain cell, or neuron, to another; that message is typically "slow down" or "stop firing." GABA tells the body when it's time to power down, and since millions of neurons in the brain respond to GABA, the effects include:

reducing anxiety

calming the nervous system

helping with sleep

relaxing the muscles.

"CBD is a GABA uptake inhibitor," says oneresearcher. "Meaning, it creates a surplus of GABA in the brain. That results in a ⬚uieting and calming effect. With CBD supplementation, patients don't have the racing thoughts that paralyze them at work or even lying awake in bed at night."

How to use CBD for anxiety?

Over the past few years, the variety of CBD products has grown exponentially. There are high CBD strains for smoking or vaping, like ACDC, Harle?uin, and Charlotte's Web. A CBD vape pen is also an option, and there are a few specifically designed to relieve anxiety, like Dosist Calm, Select Oil's CBD collection, and Aya's Relax. Edibles high in cannabidiol are another popular choice for those wishing to use CBD for anxiety, like "Not Pot" CBD-only chocolates.

But one of the most popular ways to consume cannabidiol is still through CBD oil. Some of the best CBD oils include brands like Green Roads World and Pure CBD Vapors. They are especially good for anxiety because they contain little to no THC so there's no risk of getting "high." Cannabis oil can be added to food or simply dropped straight under the tongue for sublingual absorption, which kicks in the relief fast. Not to mention, CBD oil has no lingering smell, so medicating is totally discreet.

There are literally hundreds of brands and strains of CBD on the market today. Always do your own research before deciding which brand, strain, or type (full spectrum or isolate) of CBD to go with.

High CBD strains that will help calm your anxiety

Since CBD strains are fairly new to the cannabis market, many of them are just mixes of each other. The gene pool for CBD strains is currently not as diverse as that of high-THC strains.

High CBD strains do not produce that cloudy, mental haziness or paranoia associated with THC.

1. CBD Critical Cure

CBD Critical Cure is an excellent cannabis strain. Bred by Barney's Farm Seeds, this strain is a cross between Critical Kush and a ruderalis strain. Considered indica-dominant, inhaling this flower is like taking a breath of calm ease. Producing about a 2:1 ratio of CBD to THC, most CBD Critical Cure buds feature around 11 percent CBD and 5 percent THC. The indica dominance of this strain makes it slightly sedative, which may be beneficial to those struggling to calm down on a difficult day. Consumers might experience a very slight psychoactive effect with this strain.

2. Harlequin

Harlequin is an excellent CBD strain. Featuring an almost 5:2 ratio of CBD to THC, this sativa does not generally produce a psychoactive high. Instead, Harlequin provides an ever so slightly energized and focused experience along with an easy mood uplift and anxiolytic (anti-anxiety) properties.

This unique flower has international heritage. A cross between Colombian, Thai, Swiss, and Nepalese landrace strains, the THC in Harlequin rarely exceeds 6 percent. The CBD in this flower can reach as high as 15 percent.

3. Sour Tsunami

Sour Tsunami is considered a one-to-one strain. That means that this flower tends to produce an even ratio of THC and CBD. The CBD in this bud may be slightly higher than the THC, often testing about 11 percent. THC averages about 10. A cross between Sour Diesel and New York Sour Diesel, this bud was one of the first high-CBD strains to become popular. Though some might experience some slight psychoactivity with this strain, Sour Tsunami provides a well-rounded and pleasant mood uplift.

4. Harle-tsu

Harle-tsu is a cross between the two equally famous high-CBD strains mentioned above:

Harlequin and Sour Tsunami. This flower is considered a high-CBD/low-THC strain. Harle-tsu often produces CBD levels that are almost 20 times higher than THC. Though, some phenotypes may produce more of a 1:1 ratio.

The result is a strain that produces no psychoactivity. Instead, this bud quietly eases anxiety and aids focus without really causing any noticeable change in cognitive function at all. Great for the day, this strain would be perfect for a vape break on a stressful day.

5. Stephen Hawking Kush

Stephen Hawking Kush is a cross between Harle-tsu and Sin City Kush. This strain is another one-to-one flower, often featuring about 5 percent CBD to 5 percent THC.

This flower is an excellent way to wind down without experiencing the paranoia or anxiety that is often associated with THC. Considered an indica, this bud has a relaxing

⊡uality to it, which may be beneficial to those who need to calm down during a panic.

6. Cannatonic

Cannatonic is a high CBD strain that features at least a 2:1 ratio of CBD to THC. A cross between two heavy indica strains, MK Ultra and G-13, this strain has a slight sedative ⊡uality. Like most CBD strains, Cannatonic promotes focus and may even help improve mental functioning in times of stress.

Typically, this strain expresses up to 17 percent CBD and around 6 percent THC. The higher the CBD, the less noticeable the foggy effects of THC will be.

7. ACDC

ACDC is a derivative of Cannatonic. The major difference is that this bud produces an almost 20 to 1 ratio of CBD to THC. This makes this strain more or less hemp. However, this flower can sometimes produce up to 6 percent THC. The CBD in this bud can reach a whopping 24 percent CBD.

Since CBD is a powerful anxiolytic, this strain may be particularly useful to those with more problematic anxiety disorders. ACDC does not produce a psychoactive high at all. Instead, it may provide feelings of alertness, focus, and serene mental clarity.

8. Canna-tsu

Similar to Harle-tsu, Canna-tsu is a true hybrid cross between Cannatonic and Sour Tsunami. Unlike Harle-tsu, Canna-tsu is generally considered to be a one-to-one strain. The THC in this bud might even be slightly higher than the CBD, often containing about 8 and 7 percent of each respective cannabinoid.

Chapter 12: Ways To Enhance The Anti-Anxiety Effects Of Cbd

CBD is a powerful anti-anxiety tool on its own. Yet, while many find CBD helpful, it works best when used in conjunction with therapy, nutritional, and appropriate medical support.

If you're hoping to get the most out of CBD for anxiety, here are a few ways to enhance the effects of the supplement:

1. Lavender

CBD is not the only plant compound with a calming effect.

While CBD may be unique in its ability to moderate memory and behavior, mixing it with other anxiolytic plant extracts may improve its anxiety-relieving abilities.

Research suggests that linalool, an aroma molecule most commonly found in lavender, has strong anxiolytic effects.

Some cannabis experts have suggested that combining CBD and linalool may have a beneficial and synergistic effect on anxiety.

Both CBD and lavender oil are available in tincture, oil, and capsule forms online.

2. Breathing techniques

In the midst of an anxiety attack, the body begins to produce excess amounts of the fight or flight hormone adrenaline.

This primes the body for an acute survival response.

When anxiety takes over, calming your physiology is an excellent emergency coping mechanism.

One of the fastest ways to calm your physiology is through deep breathing.

Taking a moment to consciously change your breathing patterns not only forces you to focus on something outside of your own thoughts but also helps transition the body to a calmer physical state.

3. Therapy

There is no doubt that many people feel that CBD produces genuine relief from anxiety.

However, CBD is only a helpful tool for overcoming anxiety, not a cure in and of itself.

Patients now have access to several different types of therapy that intend to create lasting relief by helping individuals change their fear patterns and behavior.

Cognitive behavioral therapy and exposure therapy are two popular forms of psychotherapy. Both types aim to help patients change patterns of thinking for an improved quality of life in the long term.

CBD FOR INSOMNIA

Insomnia is a medical condition that nearly all of us go through at some point in our lives. This can be due to a wide range of reasons. However, it is treatable. And no, we're not suggesting you start taking sleeping pills. It is widely known that sleeping pills can be harmful to the human body, especially when it becomes a habit. A lack of sex drive as well as anxiety has been observed in people who freuently use sleeping pills. CBD, on the other hand, can be the answer to all your sleeping problems as it offers the best solution.

CBD for insomnia is a great choice. This is due to CBD's ability to regulate sleep cycles, helping to decrease activity in the brain and lead you to a restful, relaxed state of mind. For those with chronic insomnia, CBD proves to be a powerful cure especially if you would prefer not to take prescription drugs or sleep aids.

The benefits of CBD for sleep

CBD is becoming a more popular choice for insomnia as sufferers from sleeplessness struggle to find a cure. For many users of CBD, better sleep is a common benefit. This is due to CBD's many positive influences on the central nervous system, including greater relaxation and mood. As CBD tends to calm anxiety and generally help with the ability to sleep soundly, this powerful, natural agent should be considered one of the best ways to sleep fully and restfully during the night.

Anti-anxiety and PTSD

PTSD is a chronic psychiatric condition, that occurs due to an emotional trauma or fear triggered in the brain and can happen to any gender or age. Studies have concluded that CBD treats all form of anxiety including post-traumatic stress disorder and anxiety-provoked sleep disorder. As CBD has anti-inflammation properties, it keeps a check on radical stress and thus helps with better sleep.

Sleep Apnea

Sleep apnea is a serious sleep disorder when your breath repeatedly starts and stops. People who suffer from sleep apnea get repeatedly awakened by their own breathing because of the narrowed airway. Therefore, you feel tired even after a snoring sleep. This can cause high blood pressure, fatigue, diabetes, etc. Studies have revealed that CBD suppresses sleep apnea, as it is a muscle relaxant.

Chronic Pain

Waking up during the night and waking early due to chronic pain is a major sleep disruption. The problems with chronic pain get worse with insomnia and sleeping disorders. CBD might be the answer to this problem as it has been found useful to treat joint pain, arthritis, back pain, etc.

Depression

Feeling sad, lack of joy, reduced interest are all symptoms of the onset of depression. It is a mood disorder that causes lack of sleep. Causes of depression can be either genetic, environmental or psychological. A chemical imbalance in the brain is also a cause of depression. According to studies, CBD restores chemical balances in the brain by releasing serotonin; that is a natural mood stabilizer.

Thousands of people have given up their sleeping pills in favor of CBD. Taking CBD oil before bed and lifestyle changes can help you with a sound sleep.

How CBD affects sleep

There are many different cannabis extracts available. CBD is just one, with THC being the other. THC, as you know, cause the psychoactive effects of the cannabis plant. For this reason, it is not the best choice for relaxation and sleep.

However, CBD actually helps with decreasing brain activity, especially at night. In one study, done in 2006, it was found that CBD helped to stimulate restfulness, but it did not cause the paranoia or overactive imagination that sometimes results from THC. CBD works by activating certain compounds in the brain, leading to a sense of peace and positive mood.

Compounds in CBD that Boost Sleep

Within CBD, there is a specific compound that actually induces sleep. Some individuals who create CBD extracts use cannabis extracts that have been aged in order to get the most benefit from CBD sleep enhancing properties. Aged CBD compounds have been shown to be the most useful at promoting good sleep.

Benefits of CBD on the Brain

For individuals suffering from pain and physical ailments, CBD can be one of the best choices for helping you fall asleep.

Through several recent studies, CBD has been shown to help alleviate symptoms of PTSD, MS, inflammation, muscular and joint dysfunction, and of course, insomnia. This is because CBD can help to relieve pain, which can prove to be a serious inhibitor of sleep. CBD can be taken as a pill or through inhaling, which is sometimes a more effective way of inducing a restful state. However, pills can act more quickly on the brain than inhalation methods, which is a consideration for those seeking a faster cure for insomnia from CBD.

CBD for Insomnia and Dreaming

Because CBD helps to create a more restful state of mind, dreaming can be better achieved through the use of this powerful agent. A study done on REM sleep while under the effect of CBD showed that users experienced more REM activity, while those who did not take cannabidiol were not able to achieve such effects.

Better Breathing withCBD

CBD has been shown to help those with asthma as well as sleep apnea. If you struggle with either of these problems, or simply can't seem to breathe soundly, regularly, and fully throughout the night, cannabidiol is a proven remedy. Some preclinical studies have shown that CBD helped over three-fourths of participants in a trial of CBD for breathing during sleep, largely due to the ability of cannabidiol to affect levels of serotonin in the brain. CBD is also able to reduce headaches and mood problems, which can also interfere with good breathing.

Improved Mood for Sleeping Soundly

One of the causes of insomnia is a racing mind or anxious thoughts while trying to fall asleep. Since CBD promotes positive mood through improved serotonin signaling as well as better dopamine levels, CBD for insomnia is undoubtedly one of the most effective ways to quickly get to sleep and stay that way. You will also find the benefits of CBD carrying through the rest of the day, in terms of better mood.

Since sound sleep can be one of the best ways to experience good moods throughout the day, CBD is considered an effective mood boosting remedy for all types of users. It is also holistic, natural, and safe, making it a good choice for those who wish to avoid non natural forms of insomnia relief.

HOW DO I TAKE CBD?

We have touched on the different ways to take CBD so far in this book. Now we're going to dive a little deeper and go into more depth. Most commonly, CBD is taken orally. This method is very easy to consume.It is discreet to use, and also it is very convenient to have a product that you can take on the go with you. In order to gain the most beneficial effects possible, you will want to look for a product that has various strains of CBD. This makes the product more potent and effective. There are many recommendations as far as dosage goes. One common method is to take 1-6mg per 10 pounds of body weight depending on your pain level. That's just a baseline. You can adjust up or down as your symptoms dictate. Although side effects are very rare, they can occur, such as dizziness, nausea or a headache. If these symptoms persist, you can stop the product or decrease the dosage. Many people experience an improvement in their symptoms after just one or two doses of CBD, but as with many products, you will find the best results occur after you have built the product up in your system a bit.

As time goes on, there is more and more research being done about CBD. Much of the findings that have already been procured, back the use of CBD as a therapeutic treatment, for many different conditions. Depending on what a person's current health status is, CBD may very well be effective in helping them lead a healthier and happier life.

It is beneficial to do your own research on CBD, rather than listening to other people's opinions. Many people are uneducated about CBD and assume it is the same thing as using marijuana or another drug. The effects of CBD are actually very beneficial and can help someone lead a very healthy life.

What steps should I take?

If you are thinking about starting up a regimen of CBD to embrace all of its potential health benefits, take some time to do your research. You'll want to think about what you want to accomplish in order to pick the right product.

Do some initial research on hemp, CBD marijuana, what are CBDs, etc. Try to learn all that you can about these products. You'll be better educated on what your options are.

It's always a good idea to talk to your doctor about CBD products. If you have been diagnosed with a medical condition of any sort, or if you are taking a prescription medication, you'll want to ensure there is no risk for interaction. Keep in mind that many medical professionals have strong opinions about cannabis in general and will not differentiate between CBD and THC or the hemp and marijuana cannabis plants.

When shopping for CBD, your best option is the internet. This is where you can find the most information, find the biggest variety of products and you have the ability to research the brands and distributors that you are considering. If you need to find out more about a potential product, contact the website or manufacturer of the product. If the lab test results on a particular brand of CBD isn't readily available on the website, don't be afraid to ask for it before you buy the product. There are many products out there that make claims that aren't true (snake oil).

After receiving a product, read the dosing information thoroughly. Make sure that you understand how to take the product, how to store the product and if there are any side effects to watch out for.

If you are thinking about increasing your dose, make sure you have waited for about three weeks before increasing the product. You'll want to wait about three weeks in between increases. This allows plenty of time for the product to build up in your system.

www.ingramcontent.com/pod-product-compliance
Lightning Source LLC
Chambersburg PA
CBHW062139020426
42335CB00013B/1262